I0482642

2012

✓SHI
School Health Index

Elementary
School

A Self-Assessment and Planning Guide

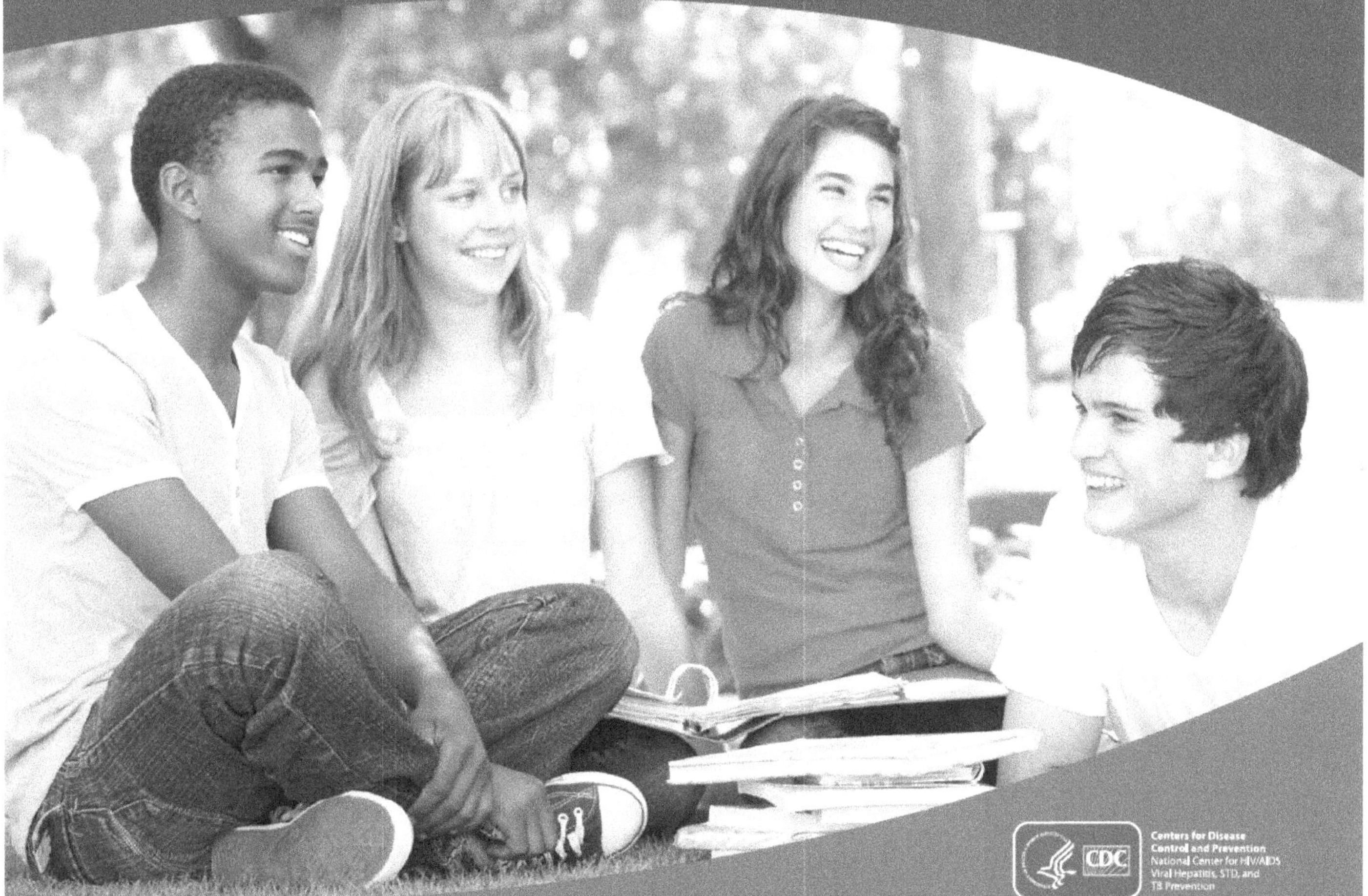

Centers for Disease Control and Prevention
National Center for HIV/AIDS
Viral Hepatitis, STD, and
TB Prevention

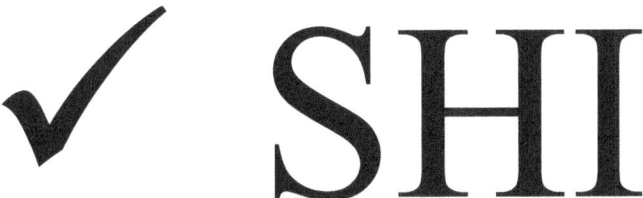

✓ SHI

School Health Index

A Self-Assessment and Planning Guide

Elementary School
2012

Contents

Suggested citation: Centers for Disease Control and Prevention. *School Health Index: A Self-Assessment and Planning Guide.* Elementary school version. Atlanta, Georgia. 2012.

Download in print or complete on CDC's website: http://www.cdc.gov/HealthyYouth/SHI/

Use of trade names and commercial sources is for identification only and does not imply endorsement by the Public Health Service or the U.S. Department of Health and Human Services.

This document was developed by the Centers for Disease Control and Prevention (CDC), National Center for HIV/AIDS, Viral Hepatitis, STD, and TB Prevention, Division of Adolescent and School Health, National Center for Chronic Disease Prevention and Health Promotion, Division of Nutrition, Physical Activity and Obesity, and Office on Smoking and Health; and the National Center for Injury Prevention and Control, Division of Unintentional Injury Prevention, and Division of Violence Prevention. Funding for the development of the first edition of the *School Health Index,* published in 2000, came from the CDC Foundation and the Robert W. Woodruff Foundation.

School Health Index Project Contributors

The following provided assistance to the development of the School Health Index. The affiliations listed are those of the contributors at the time they participated.

Jacquee Albers
New York Department of Education
Albany, NY

Maria P. Alexander, M.P.H.
Centers for Disease Control and Prevention
Atlanta, GA

Eduardo A. Alvarado, M.P.H.
Centers for Disease Control and Prevention
Atlanta, GA

Kathy M. Anderson, M.S., R.D.
North Carolina Department of Environment,
Health and Natural Resources
Raleigh, NC

Harriet Arvey, Ed.D.
Houston Independent School District
Houston, TX

Marybell Avery, Ph.D.
Lincoln Public Schools
Lincoln, NE

Kymm Ballard
North Carolina Department of Public Instruction
Raleigh, NC

Lisa C. Barrios, Sc.M., Dr.P.H.
Centers for Disease Control and Prevention
Atlanta, GA

Kim M. Boring
American Heart Association
Dallas, TX

Marilyn Briggs, M.S., R.D.
California Department of Education
Sacramento, CA

Rebekah Buckley, M.P.H., C.R.T., A.E.-C.
Centers for Disease Control and Prevention
Atlanta, GA

Charlene R. Burgeson, M.A.
Centers for Disease Control and Prevention
Atlanta, GA

Dorothy Caldwell, M.S., R.D., L.D.
U.S. Department of Agriculture Food, Nutrition and
Consumer Services
Alexandria, VA

Stephen Carey
Rhode Island Department of Education
Providence, RI

Marion W. Carter, Ph.D.
Centers for Disease Control and Prevention
Atlanta, GA

Maria Teresa Cerqueria, Ph.D., R.D.
Pan American Health Organization,
World Health Organization
Washington, DC

Lilian W. Y. Cheung, D.Sc., R.D.
Harvard School of Public Health
Boston, MA

Isobel Contento, Ph.D.
Teachers College, Columbia University
New York, NY

Carlos Crespo, Dr.P.H.
American University
Washington, DC

Peter W. Cribb, M.A., M.Ed.
University of Texas-Houston
Houston, TX

Linda Crossett, R.D.H.
Centers for Disease Control and Prevention
Atlanta, GA

Sandy A. Denham, M.A.
Muscogee County School District
Columbus, GA

Helen M. Derryberry, R.D., L.D.N.
Tennessee Department of Education
Nashville, TN

Patricia Dittus, Ph.D.
Centers for Disease Control and Prevention
Atlanta, GA

Allison M. Drury, M.P.H.
Centers for Disease Control and Prevention
Atlanta, GA

Tracey Elder
University of Georgia
Athens, GA

Sherry Everett Jones, Ph.D., M.P.H., J.D.
Centers for Disease Control and Prevention
Atlanta, GA

Diane Farr
Austin Independent School District
Austin, TX

Amy M. Fasula, Ph.D., M.P.H.
Centers for Disease Control and Prevention
Atlanta, GA

Joyce Fetro, Ph.D., C.H.E.S., F.A.S.
Southern Illinois University
Carbondale, IL

Patricia Fishback
National PTA
Brookings, SD

Carolyn Fisher, Ed.D.
Centers for Disease Control and Prevention
Atlanta, GA

Jean Forster, Ph.D.
University of Minnesota
Minneapolis, MN

Mara Galic, M.H.Sc., R.D.
Centers for Disease Control and Prevention
Atlanta, GA

Bindi Gandhi, M.A.
Centers for Disease Control and Prevention
Atlanta, GA

Alison Gardner, M.S., R.D.
Vermont Department of Health
Burlington, VT

Corinne Graffunder, M.P.H.
Centers for Disease Control and Prevention
Atlanta, GA

Brenda Z. Greene, M.F.A.
National School Boards Association
Alexandria, VA

Linda Nightingale Greenwood, M.A.
Rhode Island Department of Education
Providence, RI

Phyllis Gingiss, Dr.P.H.
University of Houston
Minneapolis, MN

Rose Haggerty, M.Ed.
Houston Independent School District
Houston, TX

Merrie Hahn
National Association of Elementary School Principals
Alexandria, VA

Lynn Hammond
South Carolina Department of Education
Columbia, SC

Samantha Harrykissoon, M.P.H.
Centers for Disease Control and Prevention
Atlanta, GA

Magdee A. Helal, Ph.D.
National Center for Educational Research and
Development
Cairo, Egypt

Carol Anne Herbert
The Valley Trust
Durban, South Africa

Albert C. Hergenroeder, M.D.
Baylor College of Medicine
Houston, TX

Marci Feldman Hertz, M.S.Ed.
Centers for Disease Control and Prevention
Atlanta, GA

James O. Hill, Ph.D.
University of Colorado Health Sciences Center
Denver, CO

Mike Hill, M.F.A.
American Cancer Society
Austin, TX

Olivia J. Hodges, Ed.D.
Gwinnett County Public Schools
Dacula, GA

Amy Hoge
American Cancer Society
Austin, TX

Pete Hunt, M.P.H., M.Ed.
Centers for Disease Control and Prevention
Atlanta, GA

Elaine Jackson, M.S.
Stewart County School System
Dover, TN

Paula Jayne, Ph.D., M.P.H.
Centers for Disease Control and Prevention
Atlanta, GA

Nina Jones
Arizona State University
Flagstaff, AZ

Christi Kay, M.Ed.
HealthMPowers, Inc.
Norcross, GA

Steven H. Kelder, Ph.D., M.P.H.
University of Texas Health Science Center
Houston, TX

Sarah Kleinman, M.P.H., C.H.E.S.
New Jersey Department of Education
Trenton, NJ

Marge Kleinsmith-Hildebrand, M.S.
San Diego Unified School District
San Diego, CA

Sarah A. Kuester, M.S., R.D.
Centers for Disease Control and Prevention
Atlanta, GA

Darrel Lang, Ed.D.
Kansas State Department of Education
Topeka, KS

Sarah Lee, Ph.D., M.S.
Centers for Disease Control and Prevention
Atlanta, GA

Sandra Leonard, R.N., M.S., F.N.P.
Centers for Disease Control and Prevention
Atlanta, GA

Nicole Liddon, Ph.D.
Centers for Disease Control and Prevention
Atlanta, GA

Penny S. Loosier, Ph.D., M.P.H.
Centers for Disease Control and Prevention
Atlanta, GA

Leslie Lytle, Ph.D., R.D.
University of Minnesota
Minneapolis, MN

Stacey Mattison, M.P.H., C.H.E.S.
Centers for Disease Control and Prevention
Atlanta, GA

Mary L. McKenna, Ph.D., R.D.
University of New Brunswick
Fredericton, New Brunswick, Canada

Thomas L. McKenzie, Ph.D.
San Diego State University
San Diego, CA

Elaine C. McLaughlin, M.S., R.D.
U.S. Department of Agriculture Food and Consumer
Service
Alexandria, VA

Aleta Mayer, Ph.D.
Virginia Commonwealth University
Richmond, VA

Sandy Nichols Mazzocco, R.N., M.Ed.
Missouri Department of Elementary and Secondary
Education
Jefferson City, MO

Tim McGloin, M.S.P.H.
University of North Carolina
Chapel Hill, NC

Sarah Merkle, M.P.H.
Centers for Disease Control and Prevention
Atlanta, GA

Caitlin Merlo, M.P.H., R.D.
Centers for Disease Control and Prevention
Atlanta, GA

Kristine M. Meurer, Ph.D.
New Mexico State Department of Education
Santa Fe, NM

Fran Anthony Meyer, Ph.D., C.H.E.S.
Society of State Directors of Health, Physical
Education and Recreation
Richmond, VA

Shannon Michael, M.P.H., Ph.D.
Centers for Disease Control and Prevention
Atlanta, GA

Linda A. Miller, M.S., R.D.
National Association of State Nutrition Education
and Training Program Coordinators
Maryland State Department of Education
Baltimore, MD

Karen Monico, M.S.
Smoking and Health Associates
Chapel Hill, NC

Nancy Murry, Dr.P.H.
University of Texas Health Science Center-Houston
Houston, TX

Patricia Nichols, M.S., C.H.E.S.
Michigan Department of Education
Lansing, MI

Guy S. Parcel, Ph.D.
University of Texas Health Science Center-Houston
Houston, TX

Russell R. Pate, Ph.D.
University of South Carolina
Columbia, SC

Carla Patterson, Ph.D.
Queensland University of Technology
Brisbane, Australia

Linda Pederson, Ph.D.
Centers for Disease Control and Prevention
Atlanta, GA

Anu Pejavara, M.P.H., C.H.E.S
Centers for Disease Control and Prevention
Atlanta, GA

Mike Penoschok, Ed.D.
Cobb County Schools,
Marietta, GA

Ruth Perou, Ph.D.
Centers for Disease Control and Prevention
Atlanta, GA

Cheryl L. Perry, Ph.D.
University of Minnesota
Minneapolis, MN

John Polomano, M.A.
Bordentown Regional School District
Bordentown, NJ

Jane Pritzl, M.A.
Centers for Disease Control and Prevention
Atlanta, GA

Alexander Prokhorov, M.D., Ph.D.
M.D. Anderson Cancer Center
Houston, TX

Neil Rainford, M.H.S.E.
Centers for Disease Control and Prevention
Atlanta, GA

Ken A. Resnicow, Ph.D.
Emory University
Atlanta, GA

Suzanne S. Rigby, M.S., R.D.
American School Food Service Association
Alexandria, VA

Leslie J. Roberts
American Association of School Administrators
Arlington, VA

Leah Robin, Ph.D.
Centers for Disease Control and Prevention
Atlanta, GA

Louise Roebke, M.S.
Redwood-Renville Counties Youth Risk Behavior
Project
Olivia, MN

Carol Runyan, M.P.H., Ph.D.
University of North Carolina
Chapel Hill, NC

Donna Sanchez, C.P.S.
New Mexico Dept. of Health
Santa Fe, NM

Spencer S. Sartorius, M.S.
Montana Office of Public Instruction
Helena, MT

Denise Seabert, Ph.D., M.C.H.E.S.
Ball State University
Muncie, IN

David Sleet, Ph.D.
Centers for Disease Control and Prevention
Atlanta, GA

Stacey Snelling, Ph.D.
American University
Washington, DC

Steve Sussman, F.A.A.H.B., Ph.D.
University of Southern California
Alhambra, CA

Don B. Sweeny, M.A.
Michigan Department of Community Health
Lansing, MI

Marlene K. Tappe, Ph.D.
Purdue University
West Lafayette, IN

Heather Tevendale, Ph.D.
Centers for Disease Control and Prevention
Atlanta, GA

Ann Kelsey Thacher, M.S.
Rhode Island Department of health
Providence, RI

Mary Thissen-Milder, Ph.D.
Minnesota Department of Children,
Families and Learning
St. Paul, MN

Debra J. Townsend
Black Hawk County Health Department
Waterloo, IA

Jackie Tselikis, R.N., M.S.Ed.
Loranger Middle School
Old Orchard Beach, ME

Carlos Vega-Matos, M.P.A.
National Association of State Boards of Education
Alexandria, VA

Mary Vernon-Smiley, M.D., M.P.H.
Centers for Disease Control and Prevention
Atlanta, GA

Stephen J. Virgilio, Ph.D.
Adelphi University
Garden City, NY

Meg Wagner, M.S., R.D., L.D.
Ohio Department of Education
Columbus, OH

D. Allan Waterfield, Ph.D.
American Cancer Society
Newark, DE

Howell Wechsler, Ed.D., M.P.H.
Centers for Disease Control and Prevention
Atlanta, GA

Lani Wheeler, M.D.
Centers for Disease Control and Prevention
Atlanta, GA

Douglas White
Wisconsin Department of Public Instruction
Madison, WI

James R. Whitehead, Ed.D.
University of North Dakota
Grand Forks, ND

Alexis M. Williams, M.P.H., C.H.E.S.
American Cancer Society
Atlanta, GA

Kristen Wolf, M.Sc.
American University
Washington, DC

Susan F. Wooley, Ph.D., C.H.E.S.
American School Health Association
Kent, OH

Judith C. Young, Ph.D.
National Association for Sport and Physical Education
Reston, VA

David Zane, M.S.
Texas Department of Health
Austin, TX

Lenore Zedosky, R.N., M.N.
West Virginia Department of Education
Charleston, WV

This page intentionally left blank.

Introduction

Why Use the School Health Index?

Promoting healthy and safe behaviors among students is an important part of the fundamental mission of schools, which is to provide young people with the knowledge and skills they need to become healthy and productive adults. Improving student health and safety can

- increase students' capacity to learn
- reduce absenteeism
- improve physical fitness and mental alertness

The School Health Index (SHI) is a self-assessment and planning guide that will enable you to

- identify the strengths and weaknesses of your school's policies and programs for promoting health and safety
- develop an action plan for improving student health and safety
- involve teachers, parents, students, and the community in improving school policies, programs, and services

There is growing recognition of the relationship between health and academic performance, and your school's results from using the SHI can help you include health promotion activities in your overall School Improvement Plan.

What Does It Involve?

The School Health Index has two activities that are to be completed by teams from your school: a self-assessment process and a planning for improvement process. The self-assessment process involves members of your school community coming together to discuss what your school is already doing to promote good health and to identify your strengths and weaknesses. More specifically, you will be assessing the extent to which your school implements the policies and practices recommended by the Centers for Disease Control and Prevention (CDC) in its research-based guidelines and strategies for school health and safety programs. The CDC School Health Guidelines are available online at www.cdc.gov/HealthyYouth.

The planning for improvement process enables you to identify recommended actions your school can take to improve its performance in areas that received low scores. It guides you through a simple process for prioritizing the various recommendations. This step will help you decide on a handful of actions to implement this year. Finally, you will complete a School Health Improvement Plan to list the steps you will take to implement your actions.

Completing the SHI is an important first step toward improving your school's health promotion policies and practices. Your school can then implement the School Health Improvement Plan and develop an ongoing process for monitoring progress and reviewing your recommendations for change. Your school's results from using the SHI can also help you include health promotion activities in your overall School Improvement Plan.

The SHI is designed for use at the school level. However, with appropriate adaptation, it could be used at the district level as well, especially if the district has only a few schools and those schools have similar policies and practices.

Should the SHI Be Used to Compare or Rate Schools?

Absolutely not! The SHI is **your** school's self-assessment tool. It is not meant to be used to compare schools. It should not be used for auditing or punishing school staff. There is no such thing as a passing grade on the SHI. You should use your SHI scores only to help you understand your school's strengths and weaknesses and to develop an action plan for improving your promotion of health and safety. Low scores on the SHI should be *expected*, and they do not indicate a "low-performing" school. They merely point you to areas in which your school can improve its health and safety promotion policies or practices.

What Resources Are Needed?

The School Health Index is available at no cost, and the assessment process for all health topics can be completed in as little as six hours. The process may take less time if fewer health topics are chosen. A small investment of time can pay big dividends in students' improved health, safety, and readiness to learn.

Many of the improvements you will want to make after completing the SHI can be done with existing staff and with few or no new resources. For those priority actions that may require new resources, your SHI results can help provide information needed to stimulate school board and community support for school health and help to establish justification to support funding requests. Some states and counties have provided financial support to cover school costs in implementing the SHI (e.g., refreshments for meetings, staff stipends) and mini-grants to help schools implement actions recommended in the School Health Improvement Plan.

What is it Based On?

The SHI is based on CDC's research-based guidelines for school health programs, which identify the policies and practices most likely to be effective in reducing youth health risk behaviors. The SHI is structured around CDC's model of coordinated school health (CSH). This model highlights the importance of involving and coordinating the efforts of all eight interactive components to maintain the well-being of young people.

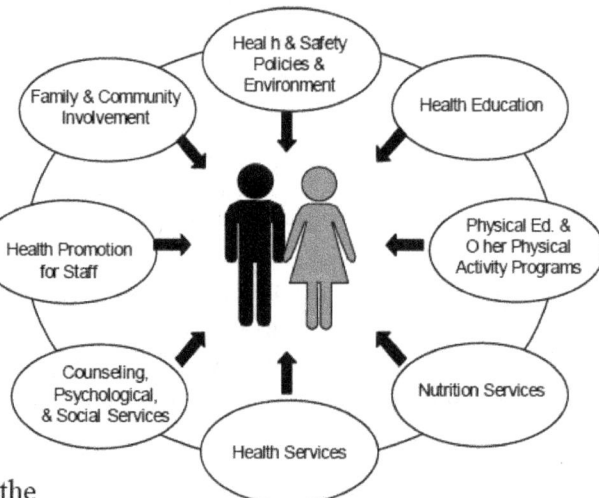

What Health Topics Does the SHI Address?

The 2012 edition of the School Health Index addresses the following health topics:

- physical activity and physical education
- nutrition
- tobacco use prevention
- asthma
- unintentional injury and violence prevention (safety)
- sexual health, including HIV, other STD and pregnancy prevention

Questions in the SHI are grouped and labeled by topic area: physical activity (PA), nutrition (N), tobacco (T), asthma (A), safety (S), sexual health (SH), and cross-cutting (CC). Cross-cutting questions address issues that are relevant to all health topics. Additionally, some questions are labeled for more than one topic (e.g., PA/S) because they are relevant to more than one (e.g., physical activity and safety). Grouping questions allows schools to choose to address some, but not all, of the health topics covered by the SHI. CDC believes that a comprehensive approach to school health is the most effective way to influence students' health behaviors. However, we recognize that some schools will want to address only one topic or just a few at a time.

Some schools have already completed the SHI for some topic areas and do not wish to revisit those questions now. Others might have funding or a mandate to address a specific health topic. The web-based version of the SHI allows you to generate score cards for specific topic areas and complete the assessment online. (Web version is available at: http://www.cdc.gov/HealthyYouth/SHI.)

Why Were These Health Topics Selected?
These topics were chosen because these health behaviors can play a critical role in preventing the leading causes of death, disability, hospitalizations, illness, and school absences and because CDC has developed guidelines or strategies for schools on addressing each of them. Additional health topics will be added in the future.

Physical inactivity, poor eating habits, and tobacco use are primary causes of the chronic diseases – such as heart disease, cancer, stroke, and diabetes – that are the leading causes of death in our nation. These risk behaviors are typically established during childhood and adolescence, and the physiological processes that lead to chronic diseases also can start in youth. Unfortunately, more children and adolescents are overweight than ever before.

Physical activity reduces the risk of premature mortality in general and of coronary heart disease, hypertension, colon cancer, and diabetes mellitus in particular. Regular physical activity in childhood and adolescence improves cardiorespiratory and muscular fitness, helps build healthy bones, helps control weight, improves cardiovascular and metabolic health biomarkers such as blood pressure and cholesterol levels, and may reduce symptoms of depression.

Nutrition involves healthy eating, which is associated with reduced risk of many diseases, including the three leading causes of death—heart disease, cancer, and stroke. Healthy eating in childhood and adolescence is important for proper growth and development and can prevent obesity, dental caries, iron deficiency anemia, and other health problems.

Tobacco use, including cigarette smoking, cigar smoking, and smokeless tobacco use, is the single leading preventable cause of death in the United States. More than one in every five high school students currently use some kind of tobacco product.

Safety relates to preventing unintentional injuries and violence, which are leading causes of death and disability among children, adolescents, and young adults. Two-thirds of all deaths among adolescents are due to either unintentional injuries or violence. Major causes of unintentional injuries include motor-vehicle crashes, drowning, poisoning, fires and burns, falls, sports- and recreation-related injuries, firearm-related injuries, choking, suffocation, and animal bites. Types of violence are homicide, suicide, assault, sexual violence, rape, child maltreatment, dating and domestic violence, and self-inflicted injuries. Children and adolescents engage in many behaviors that increase their risk of injury, including not using seat belts, driving after drinking alcohol, carrying weapons, and engaging in physical fights.

Asthma is a prevalent chronic respiratory disease characterized by periodic episodes of increased inflammation and narrowing of the small airways. Symptoms may include wheezing, coughing, chest tightness, and difficulty breathing. Asthma is among the leading causes of hospitalizations and a leading cause of school absences. On average, in a classroom of 30 children, about three are likely to have asthma. The impact of illness and deaths due to asthma is disproportionately higher among low-income populations, minorities, and children in inner cities than in the general population. Asthma cannot be cured, but it can be controlled. Schools can do their part to control asthma by becoming more "asthma-friendly"– that is, by adopting policies and procedures and coordinating student services to better serve students with asthma.

Sexual risk behaviors place adolescents at risk for HIV infection, other sexually transmitted diseases (STD), and unintended pregnancy. Many young people engage in sexual risk behaviors that can result in unintended health outcomes. Nearly half of all U.S. high school students have had sexual intercourse. Nearly half of the 19 million new STD acquired each year are among young people aged 15–24 years.

Instructions for Site Coordinator

There is no single way to implement the SHI. Schools have developed many approaches and you need to find the approach that meets your school's needs. The most essential thing to remember is that completing the SHI should be a group effort: the strength of the process comes from having individuals from different parts of the school community sit down together and plan ways to work towards improving school policies and programs. The connections that develop among SHI participants are among the most important outcomes of the process.

You can complete the SHI online or follow the step-by-step instructions below to complete the print version. Both methods are effective and you need to decide which one is best for your school. The online method is interactive and customizable. You can select the topics you want to include in your SHI and invite your team members to log in and participate. Access the SHI online at http://www.cdc.gov/HealthyYouth/SHI.

Step-by-Step Instructions

1. **Review the eight modules.** Habits and practices related to health and safety are influenced by the entire school environment. That's why the SHI has eight different modules that correspond to the eight components of coordinated school health (See Introduction or www.cdc.gov/HealthyYouth/cshp.)

2. **Assemble the School Health Index team.** Identify a team of people who will be responsible for completing the SHI. You may choose to create a new team; use an existing team, such as the school health council; or create a new subcommittee of the school management council. Broad and diverse participation is important for meaningful assessment and successful planning and implementation.

   Below are key people who you may want to invite to join the SHI team. Choose people you think are appropriate to represent your school and community.

   - Principal, Assistant Principal
   - Physical education teacher
   - Health education teacher
   - Classroom teacher
   - Student
   - School nutrition services manager
   - Athletic coach
   - School counselor, psychologist or social worker
   - School nurse or health care provider
   - School security personnel
   - Bus driver
   - Janitor or custodial worker
   - Facility and maintenance staff
   - Parent or other family member
   - Community-based health care and social services provider
   - Community health organization representative, e.g., American Cancer Society
   - Local health department staff member

   Getting support for the use of the SHI from school administrators greatly improves overall commitment to completing the SHI and implementing the School Health Improvement Plan. School and district-level administrators can give the SHI team the power to implement identified changes.

3. **Identify a coordinator for the School Health Index team.** The identity of the SHI coordinator varies from school to school. Many schools have found that it is best to have someone from outside the school facilitate the SHI process. This person might be, for example, a retired health educator, a community-based dietitian, a professor at a local university, a graduate student, or a volunteer at a community-based health organization. Because they are removed from school politics, these individuals are neutral and can help the staff deal with internal conflicts. A SHI coordinator should be
   - a skilled group facilitator who can keep meeting participants on task while making them feel good about their participation
   - an excellent listener who does not attempt to impose his or her own opinions on the group
   - an individual who is highly respected by all participants and by the school administration

4. **Meet with all members of the SHI team.**
   - Explain the SHI and its purposes. Use the resources, including PowerPoint presentations, provided in the SHI Training Manual to help plan this meeting. (See http://www.cdc.gov/HealthyYouth/SHI/training.)
   - Encourage team members to answer all questions as accurately as possible. Team members should understand that results will not be used for punishing schools or comparing your school to other schools.
   - Make sure that all team members understand that their work on the SHI can make a great difference in the lives of your school's students. Completing the SHI is not an academic exercise or a bureaucratic mandate; it is a process for bringing people together to improve a school's policies and programs.

5. **Complete the self-assessment process.** Decide whether you want to use the online version or the paper version. If you decide to complete the SHI online, create an account and a SHI for your team. After creating the account, distribute the login information to the team members. Members of your team can log into the system at any time by using the account information to answer the discussion questions assigned to them or to perform other tasks.

   Decide how you want to complete the SHI self-assessment process. Some schools have their entire SHI team stay together to do the entire self-assessment, sometimes in just one meeting. Others form sub-teams of two or more people to work on each of the eight modules. It is very important to have at least two people work on each module, because having more than one person involved will increase accuracy and elicit a variety of creative insights for improving school policies and programs.

   Answer the discussion questions. Read through the questions carefully and select the answer that best describes your school. Words and phrases that are **underlined and bolded** are further defined in the SHI Glossary. Clicking on these words in the online version will take you directly to this additional information. If a question does not apply to your school, you can designate it as not applicable. If you are not sure or need more information before you can answer the question, you can skip it and return to it at another time. You do not have to answer all the questions in a module.

Whoever completes the paper version of the modules will need to receive copies of the following documents:

- Instructions for module coordinator
- Module Score Card and Sample Completed Module Score Card
- Module Discussion Questions
- Module Planning Questions and Sample Completed Planning Questions
- SHI Glossary

Individuals working on each module need to

- answer the module Discussion Questions by writing the results on the module Score Card
- review the module Score Card results to answer the module Planning Questions
- use the results from the third Planning Question to identify the one, two, or three highest priority actions for this module that will be recommended for implementation this year

For some modules this will take just minutes, but for others it may take an hour or more.

6. **Complete the Overall Score Card.** Collect the Score Cards for each module, and transfer the scores to the Overall Score Card (located in the Planning for Improvement section). Make copies of the completed Overall Score Card for every SHI team member.

7. **Meet with all SHI team members to review score cards and create your School Health Improvement Plan.** Use the resources provided in the SHI Training Manual to help plan this second meeting. (See http://www.cdc.gov/HealthyYouth/SHI/training.)
   - Review the Score Cards for each module. Discuss the identified strengths and weaknesses and recommended actions in each module.
   - Review the Overall Score Card.
   - Have all participants work together to identify the top priority actions for the entire school.
   - Complete the School Health Improvement Plan (located in the Planning for Improvement section). This involves setting 3 to 5 priority actions, discussing the resources needed and action steps, assigning responsibilities, setting timelines, and deciding how to present the plan to the school leadership and community.
   - Discuss how you will monitor progress and when the team will meet again.

WHAT DO WE DO IF A QUESTION SEEMS IRRELEVANT FOR OUR SCHOOL?
It is possible that some questions might not be relevant for every school. If you are sure that this is the case, you may choose not to answer the question. If you are using the paper version of the SHI just remember to appropriately adjust the denominator used for calculating the Overall Module Score (i.e., subtract 3 points for each question deleted).

In many cases questions that might appear to be irrelevant can be re-interpreted to become relevant. For example, a question might ask about the school's gymnasium or cafeteria, and your school might not have a gymnasium or cafeteria. However, if students participate in physical education or eat meals somewhere on campus, you can modify the question to make it fit your circumstances. If meals are cooked off-site at a central cooking facility, it might be harder for you to obtain information about food preparation practices and to influence those practices – but it can be done. Planning Question 3 will ask you to consider feasibility. Trying to influence practices at a central cooking facility might not be a high priority for your school because it might rate low on feasibility.

This page intentionally left blank.

Sample Completed Score Card
Module 1: School Health and Safety Policies and Environment

Instructions

1. Carefully read and discuss the Module 1 Discussion Questions (pages 5-28), which contains questions and scoring descriptions for each item listed on this Score Card.
2. Circle the most appropriate score for each item.
3. After all questions have been scored, calculate the overall Module Score and complete the Module 1 Planning Questions located at the end of this module (pages 29-30).

		Fully in Place	Partially in Place	Under Develop-ment	Not in Place
CC.1	Representative school health committee or team	3	2	1	0
CC.2	Written school health and safety policies	3	2	1	0
CC.3	Communicate health and safety policies to students, parents, staff members, and visitors	3	2	1	0
CC.4	Positive school climate	3	2	1	0
CC.5	Overcome barriers to learning	3	2	1	0
CC.6	Enrichment experiences	3	2	1	0
CC.7	Local wellness policies	3	2	1	0
CC.8	Standard precautions policy	3	2	1	0
CC.9	Professional development on meeting diverse needs of students	3	2	1	0
CC.10	Prevent harassment and bullying	3	2	1	0
CC.11	Active supervision	3	2	1	0
CC.12	Written crisis response plan	3	2	1	0
PA.1	Recess	3	2	1	0
PA.2	Access to physical activity facilities outside school hours	3	2	1	0
PA.3	Adequate physical activity facilities	3	2	1	0
PA.4	Prohibit using physical activity as punishment	3	2	1	0
N.1	Prohibit using food as reward or punishment	3	2	1	0
N.2	Access to free drinking water	3	2	1	0
N.3	All foods offered or sold during the school day meet strong nutrition standards	3	2	1	0
N.4	All beverages offered or sold during the school day meet strong nutrition standards	3	2	1	0
N.5	Fundraising efforts during and outside school hours meet strong nutrition standards	3	2	1	0
N.6	Advertising and promotion of foods and beverages	3	2	1	0
N.7	Hands washed before meals and snacks	3	2	1	0
COLUMN TOTALS: For each column, add up the numbers that are circled and enter the sum in this row.		24	18	5	0

(If you decide to skip any of the topic areas, make sure you adjust the denominator for the Module Score (69) by subtracting 3 for each question eliminated).

TOTAL POINTS: Add the four sums above and enter the total to the right.	47

NOTE! For simplicity, this example shows only Cross-Cutting, Physical Activity, and Nutrition Items. The denominator has been adjusted accordingly.

MODULE SCORE = (Total Points / **69**) X 100	68%

Sample Completed Planning Questions
Module 1: School Policies and Environment

The Module 1 Planning Questions will help your school use its School Health Index results to identify and prioritize changes that will improve policies and programs to improve students' health and safety.

Planning Question 1
Look back at the scores you assigned to each question. According to these scores, what are the **strengths** and the **weaknesses** of your school's policies and environment related to students' health and safety?

Strengths
- Excellent communication of policies with parents, visitors, and staff.
- Offer a wide variety of enrichment experiences.
- Students are actively supervised.
- Have a strong standard precautions policy.
- Do not use physical activity as punishment.
- Free drinking water is widely available and students can bring bottles to class.
- Students are given enough time to wash their hands before eating.

Weaknesses
- Do not have a committee to oversee our health programs (CC.1).
- Local wellness policy has not been implemented at the school level (CC.7).
- Could improve our support for students who have been bullied (CC.10).
- Recess is not provided every day (PA.1).
- Some teachers still use candy as rewards (N.1).
- Some food available during the school day does not meet strong nutrition standards (N.3).

Planning Question 2
For each of the weaknesses identified above, list several recommended actions to improve the school's scores (e.g., create and maintain a school health committee).

1. Form a school health committee.
2. Have the school health committee review the district local wellness policy.
3. Conduct staff development on dealing with bullying.
4. Make sure all teachers are providing daily, 20 minute recess.
5. Give teachers ideas about non-candy rewards.
6. Work with the nutrition services staff to make sure all foods meet strong nutrition standards.

SCHOOL HEALTH INDEX – ELEMENTARY SCHOOL

Planning Question 3. List each of the actions identified in Planning Question 2 on the table below. Use the five-point scales defined below to score each action on five dimensions (importance, cost, time, commitment, feasibility). Add the points for each action to get the total points. Use the total points to help you choose one, two, or three top priority actions that you will recommend to the School Health Index team for implementation this year.

Importance	**How important is the action?**		
	5 = Very important	3 = Moderately important	1 = Not important
Cost	**How expensive would it be to plan and implement the action?**		
	5 = Not expensive	3 = Moderately expensive	1 = Very expensive
Time	**How much time and effort would it take to implement the action?**		
	5 = Little or no time and effort	3 = Moderate time and effort	1 = Very great time and effort
Commitment	**How enthusiastic would the school community be about implementing the action?**		
	5 = Very enthusiastic	3 = Moderately enthusiastic	1 = Not enthusiastic
Feasibility	**How difficult would it be to attain the action?**		
	5 = Not difficult	3 = Moderately difficult	1 = Very difficult

Module 1 Actions	Importance	Cost	Time	Commitment	Feasibility	Total Points	Top Priority Action?
Form a school health committee.	5	5	4	3	3	20	✓
Have the school health committee review the district local wellness policy.	3	5	2	2	4	16	
Conduct staff development on dealing with bullying.	5	3	3	5	4	20	✓
Make sure all teachers are providing daily, 20 minute recess.	4	5	4	3	4	20	✓
Give teachers ideas about non-candy rewards.	3	5	3	2	3	16	
Work with the nutrition services staff to make sure all foods meet strong nutrition standards.	3	2	2	2	2	12	

This page intentionally left blank.

Module 1: School Health and Safety Policies and Environment

Instructions for Module Coordinator

Habits and practices related to health and safety are influenced by the entire school environment. That's why the School Health Index has eight different modules, which correspond to the eight components of coordinated school health in the figure below.

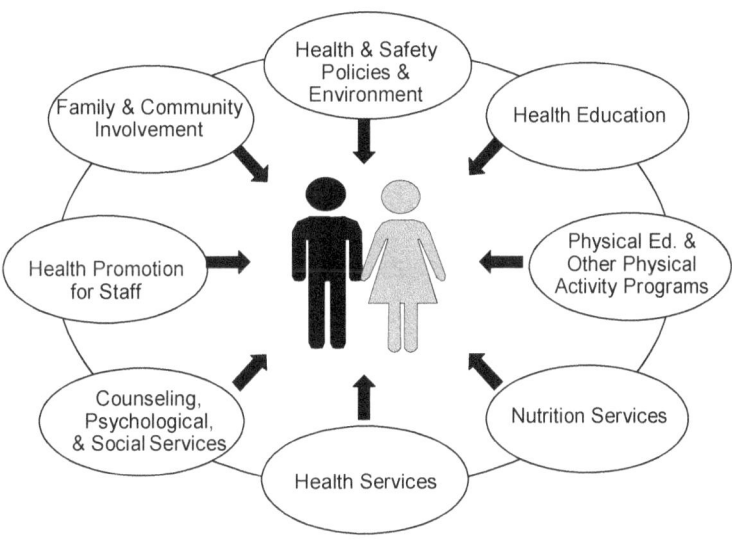

Instructions for completing the module

1. Work with the site coordinator to organize a team to complete the module's documents. Below are some suggested members of the Module 1 team.

Principal	Parent(s)
Assistant principal	Student(s)
School nutrition services manager	School nurse or health care provider
Physical education teacher(s)	Community health agency representative(s)
Health education teacher(s)	(e.g., American Cancer Society, local health
School security personnel	department)
School psychologist	School social worker
Other teacher(s)	

2. Make a photocopy of the module Discussion Questions (pages 5-27) for each Module 1 team member. Make at least one photocopy of the module Score Card (pages 3-4) and the module Planning Questions (pages 29-30).

3. Give each Module 1 team member a copy of the Module 1 Discussion Questions. Use the copies of the module Score Card and the Planning Questions to record the team's work. Put the originals of these documents aside in case you need to make more photocopies.

4. At a Module 1 team meeting:

    - Discuss each of the Module 1 Discussion Questions and its scoring choices.
    - Decide how to collect any information you need to answer each question accurately.
    - After you have all the information you need, arrive at a consensus score for each question. Answer each question as accurately as possible. The SHI is **your** self-assessment tool for identifying strengths and weaknesses and for planning improvements; it should not be used for evaluating staff.
    - Record the scores (0-3) for each question on the module Score Card and calculate the overall Module Score.
    - Use the scores written on the module Score Card to complete the Planning Questions at the end of the module.
    - Use the results from the third Planning Question to identify the one, two, or three highest priority actions that you will recommend to the SHI team for implementation this year.
    - Use the answers to the Planning Questions to decide how you will present your results and recommendations at the follow-up SHI team meeting.

We wish you success in your efforts to improve the health and safety of young people!

Module 1: School Health and Safety Policies and Environment
Score Card

Instructions

3. Carefully read and discuss the Module 1 Discussion Questions (pages 5-27), which contains questions and scoring descriptions for each item listed on this Score Card.
4. Circle the most appropriate score for each item.
3. After all questions have been scored, calculate the overall Module Score and complete the Module 1 Planning Questions located at the end of this module (pages 29-30).

		Fully in Place	Partially in Place	Under Develop-ment	Not in Place
CC.1	Representative school health committee or team	3	2	1	0
CC.2	Written school health and safety policies	3	2	1	0
CC.3	Communicate health and safety policies to students, parents, staff members, and visitors	3	2	1	0
CC.4	Positive school climate	3	2	1	0
CC.5	Overcome barriers to learning	3	2	1	0
CC.6	Enrichment experiences	3	2	1	0
CC.7	Local wellness policies	3	2	1	0
CC.8	Standard precautions policy	3	2	1	0
CC.9	Professional development on meeting diverse needs of students	3	2	1	0
CC.10	Prevent harassment and bullying	3	2	1	0
CC.11	Active supervision	3	2	1	0
CC.12	Written crisis response plan	3	2	1	0
S.1	Safe physical environment	3	2	1	0
S.2	Maintain safe physical environment	3	2	1	0
S.3	Staff development on unintentional injuries, violence, and suicide	3	2	1	0
PA.1	Recess	3	2	1	0
PA.2	Access to physical activity facilities outside school hours	3	2	1	0
PA.3	Adequate physical activity facilities	3	2	1	0
PA.4	Prohibit using physical activity as punishment	3	2	1	0
N.1	Prohibit using food as reward or punishment	3	2	1	0
N.2	Access to free drinking water	3	2	1	0
N.3	All foods offered or sold during the school day meet strong nutrition standards	3	2	1	0
N.4	All beverages offered or sold during the school day meet strong nutrition standards	3	2	1	0
N.5	Fundraising efforts during and outside school hours meet strong nutrition standards	3	2	1	0
N.6	Advertising and promotion of foods and beverages	3	2	1	0
N.7	Hands washed before meals and snacks	3	2	1	0
T.1	Prohibit tobacco use among students	3	2	1	0
T.2	Prohibit tobacco use among school staff members and visitors	3	2	1	0
T.3	Enforce tobacco-use policies	3	2	1	0
T.4	Prohibit tobacco advertising	3	2	1	0
A.1	Written policies for carry and self-administration of quick-relief medications	3	2	1	0
A.2	Professional development on asthma	3	2	1	0
A.3	Implement indoor air quality practices	3	2	1	0

A.4	Implement integrated pest management practices	3	2	1	0
SH.1	Non-discrimination on the basis of HIV infection policy	3	2	1	0
SH.2	Confidentiality of HIV status	3	2	1	0
SH.3	Professional development for all staff members on HIV policies or laws	3	2	1	0
SH.4	Professional development for administrators and teachers on HIV, other STD, and pregnancy prevention	3	2	1	0

COLUMN TOTALS: For each column, add up the numbers that are circled and enter the sum in this row.

(If you decide to skip any of the topic areas, make sure you adjust the denominator for the Module Score (114) by subtracting 3 for each question eliminated).

TOTAL POINTS: Add the four sums above and enter the total to the right.

MODULE SCORE =
(Total Points / 114) X 100   %

Module 1: School Health and Safety Policies and Environment

Discussion Questions

CC.1 Representative school health committee or team

Does your school have a **representative** committee or team that meets at least four times a year and oversees school health and safety **policies** and programs?

3 = Yes.
2 = There is a committee or team that does this, **but** it could be more representative.
1 = There is a committee or team, but it is **not** representative, **or** it meets less often than four times a year.
0 = No.

CC.2 Written school health and safety policies

Does your school or district have written health and safety **policies** that include the following components?
✓ Rationale for developing and implementing the policy
✓ Population for which the policy applies (e.g., students, staff, visitors)
✓ Where the policy applies (e.g., on or off school property)
✓ When the policy applies
✓ Programs supported by the policy
✓ Designation of person(s) responsible (e.g., school administrator(s), teachers) for implementing the policy
✓ Designation of person(s) responsible (e.g., school administrator(s), teachers) for enforcing the policy
✓ Communication procedures (e.g., through staff meetings, **professional development**, website, staff handbook) of the policy
✓ Procedures for addressing policy infractions
✓ Definitions of terms

3 = **All** of our health and safety policies include **all** of these components.
2 = **Most** of our health and safety policies include **all** of these components.
1 = **Some** of our health and safety policies include **some** of these components.
0 = **Few** of our health and safety policies include only a **few** of these components, **or** our school or district does **not** have any health and safety policies.

CC.3 Communicate health and safety policies to students, parents, staff members, and visitors

Does your school communicate its school or district health and safety **policies** in all of the following ways?
- ✓ Signs (e.g., tobacco-free, weapon-free)
- ✓ Staff member orientation
- ✓ Staff meetings
- ✓ Student orientation
- ✓ Student handbook
- ✓ Staff handbook or listserv
- ✓ Employee contracts
- ✓ Parent handbook, newsletters, or listserv
- ✓ Policies included in contracts with outside vendors and organizations that use school facilities
- ✓ Announcements at school events
- ✓ School-sponsored meetings
- ✓ Community meetings
- ✓ School or district website

3 = Yes, in **all** of these ways.
2 = In **most** of these ways.
1 = In **some** of these ways.
0 = In **none** of these ways.

CC.4 Positive School Climate

Does your school foster a **positive psychosocial school climate** using all of the following practices?

✓ Communicate clear expectations for learning and behavior to students, and share those expectations with families to encourage them to reinforce them at home
✓ Foster pro-social behavior by engaging students in activities such as peer tutoring, classroom chores, service learning, and teacher assistance
✓ Foster an appreciation of student and family diversity and respect for all families' cultural beliefs and practices
✓ Hold school-wide activities that give students opportunities to learn about diverse cultures and experiences
✓ Use instructional materials that reflect the diversity of your student body
✓ Challenge **staff members** to greet each student by name
✓ Expect staff members to encourage students to ask for help when needed
✓ Expect staff members to take timely action to solve problems reported by students or parents
✓ Expect staff members to praise positive student behavior to students and their parents

3 = Yes, our school fosters a positive psychosocial school climate by using **all** of these practices.
2 = Our school fosters a positive psychosocial school climate by using **most** of these practices.
1 = Our school fosters a positive psychosocial school climate by using **some** of these practices.
0 = Our school does **not** foster a positive psychosocial school climate by using these practices.

CC.5 Overcome barriers to learning

Does your school offer, to all students who need them, a variety of services designed to help students overcome **barriers to learning**?

3 = Yes.
2 = Our school offers a variety of services to **most** but not to all students who need them.
1 = Our school offers a limited variety of services, **or** many students who need them do not have access to them.
0 = No, our school does **not** offer such services.

CC.6 Enrichment experiences

Does your school provide a broad variety of student **enrichment experiences** that are accessible to all students?

3 = Yes.
2 = Our school offers a variety of experiences, **but** some students do not have access to them.
1 = Our school offers a limited variety of experiences, **or** many students do not have access to them.
0 = No, our school does **not** offer enrichment experiences.

CC.7 Local Wellness Policies

Has your school <u>implemented</u> the following components of the district's local wellness policy?
- ✓ Nutrition education activities
- ✓ Physical activity opportunities
- ✓ Guidelines for reimbursable school meals which are as strong as or stronger than federal regulations
- ✓ Nutrition guidelines for all foods available on the school campus during the school day that promote student health and reduce childhood obesity
- ✓ Other school-based activities that promote student wellness
- ✓ Involvement of parents, students, school **staff members**, administrators, and the general public in policy development, implementation, periodic review and updates
- ✓ Regular reporting on content and implementation to the public (including parents, students, and community members)
- ✓ Periodic measurement of school compliance with the local wellness policy and progress updates made available to the public
- ✓ Designation of a lead school official to ensure compliance with local wellness policy

NOTE: By the start of the 2006-2007 school year, every school district participating in the federal meal program was required to establish a local school wellness policy. This requirement was updated in 2010 placing greater emphasis on evaluation and sharing progress of local wellness policy implementation with the public. Your school health team should review your district's policy before completing this question.

3 = Yes, our school has implemented **all** of these components.
2 = Our school has implemented **most** of these components.
1 = Our school has implemented a **few** of these components.
0 = No, we have **not** implemented any of these components, **or** our policy does not include any of these components, **or** our district does not have a local wellness policy.

CC.8 Standard precautions policy

Does your school implement a **standard precautions** policy that includes all of the following components?
- ✓ Providing and requiring the use of latex or poly gloves and eye wear when exposed to blood and body fluids
- ✓ Providing a hard-sided container for contaminated needles/sharps in offices where syringes may be used
- ✓ Appropriate disinfecting of surface areas and clean-up materials after exposure to blood and body fluid
- ✓ Instructions for appropriate disposal of contaminated materials (e.g., dressings, clothing, tissue/towels)
- ✓ Procedures and follow-up for **staff members** who are exposed to blood

3 = Yes, our school implements a standard precautions policy that includes all **five** of these components.

2 = Our school implements a standard precautions policy that includes **three or four** of these components.

1 = Our school implements a standard precautions policy that includes **one or two** of these components.

0 = Our school's standard precautions policy does **not** include any of these components, or we do not have a standard precautions policy.

CC.9 Professional development on meeting diverse needs of students

Have all teachers received **professional development** on **meeting the diverse cognitive, emotional, and social needs** of children and adolescents in the past two years?

3 = Yes, **all** teachers have received professional development on ways to meet the diverse needs of children and adolescents.

2 = **Most** teachers have received professional development on ways to meet the diverse needs of children and adolescents.

1 = **Some** teachers have received professional development on ways to meet the diverse needs of children and adolescents.

0 = **No** teachers have received professional development on ways to meet the diverse needs of children and adolescents.

CC.10   Prevent harassment and bullying

Has the school established a climate, in each of the following ways, that prevents **harassment** and **bullying**?
- ✓ **Staff members**, students and parents are informed through a variety of mechanisms of **policies** defining harassment and bullying and explaining the consequences of such behaviors
- ✓ Disciplinary policies are fairly and consistently implemented among all student groups
- ✓ Staff members and students treat each other with respect and courtesy
- ✓ Fair play and nonviolence is emphasized on the playground, on the school bus, and at school events
- ✓ Students are encouraged to report harassment or bullying, including through anonymous reporting methods
- ✓ Support is provided for victims of harassment or bullying

3 = Yes, in each of these **five** ways.
2 = In **four** of these ways.
1 = In **three** of these ways.
0 = In **two or fewer** of these ways.

CC.11   Active supervision

Do **staff members actively supervise** students, in each of the following ways, everywhere on campus (e.g., classroom, lunchroom, playground, locker room, hallways, bathroom, and school bus)?
- ✓ Observing students and being available to talk to students before, during, and after school
- ✓ Anticipating and effectively responding to unsafe situations
- ✓ Discouraging pushing and **bullying**
- ✓ Promoting prosocial behaviors, such as cooperation, conflict resolution, and helping others

3 = Yes, in each of these **four** ways.
2 = In **three** of these ways.
1 = In **two** of these ways.
0 = In **one or none** of these ways.

CC.12 Written crisis response plan

Does your school have a written **crisis response plan** that includes preparedness, response, and recovery elements? Is the plan practiced regularly and updated as necessary?

3 = Yes, our school has a written crisis response plan that includes preparedness, response, and recovery efforts, **and** it is practiced and updated regularly.

2 = Our school's plan includes preparedness and response, **but** not recovery elements, and it is practiced and updated regularly.

1 = Our school's plan does **not** include all the necessary components, **or** it is not practiced regularly, **or** it is not updated as necessary.

0 = We do **not** have a written crisis response plan.

S.1   Safe physical environment

Does the school provide a safe physical environment, inside and outside school buildings, by following all of these practices?
✓ Flooring surfaces are slip-resistant and stairways have sturdy guardrails
✓ Poisons and chemical hazards are labeled and are stored in locked cabinets
✓ First-aid equipment and notices describing safety procedures are available
✓ All areas of the school have sufficient lighting, and secluded areas are sealed off or supervised
✓ Smoke alarms, sprinklers, and fire extinguishers are installed and operational
✓ Pedestrians are offered special protection, including crossing guards, escorts, crosswalks, and safe bus and car loading
✓ A variety of methods are used to keep weapons out of the school environment
✓ School buses do not idle while loading or unloading students, to reduce emission of diesel exhaust and fine particles
✓ Spaces and facilities for physical activity (including playgrounds and sports fields) meet or exceed recommended safety standards
✓ The campus and buildings are pleasant and welcoming (e.g., uncluttered, uncrowded, well-lit, graffiti-free)

3 = Yes, **all** of these practices are followed.
2 = All the safety practices are followed, **but** at times the school has temporary lapses in one of them.
1 = One of the safety practices is **not** followed, **or** at times the school has temporary lapses in more than one of them.
0 = More than one of the safety practices are **not** followed.

S.2   Maintain safe physical environment

Does the school maintain a safe physical environment by following all of these practices?
✓ Conduct annual comprehensive safety assessment and monthly assessment of playgrounds and sports fields
✓ Each day players and coaches walk the sports field to ensure that it is free of potholes, glass, and other safety hazards
✓ Designate one person with the responsibility for addressing hazards
✓ Designate a clear procedure for reporting hazards to the responsible person
✓ Make repairs immediately after hazards have been identified

3 = Yes, **all** of these practices are followed.
2 = All the practices are followed, **but** assessments are done less frequently than stated.
1 = One of the maintenance practices is **not** followed.
0 = More than one of the maintenance practices are **not** followed.

S.3 Staff development on unintentional injuries, violence, and suicide

Have all **staff members** received **professional development** on preventing unintentional injuries, violence, and suicide in the past 2 years?

3 = Yes, **all** have.
2 = **Most** have.
1 = **Some** have.
0 = **None** have.

PA.1 Recess

Are students provided at least 20 minutes of **recess** during each school day, and do teachers or recess monitors encourage students to be active?

NOTE: Recess should complement **physical education** class, not substitute for it.

3 = Yes.
2 = Recess is provided for at least 20 minutes each day, **but** teachers or recess monitors do not encourage students to be active.
1 = Recess is provided each day but for less than 20 minutes, **or** it is provided on some days but not on all days.
0 = Recess is **not** provided on any day.

PA.2 Access to physical activity facilities outside school hours

Can all students use your school's indoor and outdoor physical activity facilities **outside school hours**?

NOTE: Use of indoor facilities should be supervised.

3 = Yes, **both** indoor and outdoor facilities are available to all students.
2 = Indoor or outdoor facilities, but **not both**, are available to all students.
1 = Indoor or outdoor facilities are available to all students, **but** the hours of availability are very limited.
0 = No, **neither** indoor nor outdoor facilities are available to all students.

PA.3 Adequate physical activity facilities

Are your physical activity facilities adequate in all of the following ways?
✓ Both indoor and outdoor spaces can be used by **physical education** classes, **intramural programs or physical activity clubs**, and **interscholastic sports** programs
✓ Indoor facilities exist so that physical education classes do not have to be canceled due to weather extremes (e.g., rain or temperatures extremes)
✓ In physical education classes, all students can be physically active without overcrowding or safety risks
✓ Facilities are accessible for persons with disabilities
✓ For physical activity clubs and interscholastic sports, all interested students can sign up and participate without overcrowding or safety risks

3 = Yes, in all **five** of these ways.
2 = In **four** of these ways.
1 = In **three** of these ways.
0 = In **two or fewer** of these ways.

PA.4 Prohibit using physical activity as punishment

Does your school prohibit using physical activity and withholding **physical education** class as **punishment**? Is this prohibition consistently followed?

NOTE: Please do not consider issues related to participation in **interscholastic sports** programs when answering this question.

3 = Yes, using physical activity as punishment and withholding physical education class as punishment are prohibited, and both prohibitions are consistently followed.
2 = One of these practices is prohibited, and this prohibition is consistently followed.
1 = One or both of these practices is prohibited, but this prohibition is not consistently followed.
0 = Neither practice is prohibited.

N.1 Prohibit using food as reward or punishment

Does your school prohibit giving students food as a reward and withholding food as **punishment**? Is this prohibition consistently followed?

3 = Yes, using food as a reward and withholding food as punishment are prohibited, and both prohibitions are consistently followed.
2 = One of these practices is prohibited, and this prohibition is consistently followed.
1 = One or both of these practices is prohibited, but this prohibition is not consistently followed.
0 = Neither practice is prohibited.

N.2 Access to free drinking water

Does your school make safe, unflavored, drinking water available throughout the school day at no cost to students?

3 = Yes, students can access water fountains or water filling stations throughout the school day, **and** they are allowed to bring filled containers to class.
2 = Students can access water fountains or water filling stations throughout the school day, but they are **not** allowed to bring filled containers to class.
1 = Students have **limited** access to water fountains or water filling stations throughout the school day.
0 = No, students do **not** have access to free, safe, unflavored, drinking water.

N.3 All foods offered or sold during the school day meet strong nutrition standards

Do all foods offered or sold during the school day outside the federal meal program (i.e., **competitive foods**) align with the criteria recommended by the Institute of Medicine's Nutrition Standards for Foods in Schools (see criteria below)?

Nutrition Standards for Foods in Schools (Elementary) for Question N.3	
All foods meet these criteria	Examples
FOODS/SNACKS ARE LIMITED TO • Fruits or vegetables (e.g., fresh, canned, dried) • Whole grain snacks • Combination snacks (e.g., made of fruit and whole grain) • Nonfat and **low-fat** dairy products FOODS/SNACKS ALSO MUST BE • ≤200 calories • ≤35% total calories from fat • <10% of calories from saturated fats • Trans fat-free • ≤35% calories from total sugars • ≤200 mg of sodium ENTREE ITEMS ARE • National School Lunch Program (NSLP) menu items • ≤35% total calories from fat • <10% of calories from saturated fats • Trans fat-free • ≤35% calories from total sugars • Have a sodium content of 480 mg or less	• Individual fruits (apples, pears, oranges) • Fruit cups packed in juice or water • Vegetables (baby carrots, broccoli, edamame) • Dried or dehydrated fruits (raisins, apricots, cherries) • 100% fruit juice or low-sodium 100% vegetable juice • Low-fat, low-salt, whole-grain crackers or chips • Whole-grain, low-sugar cereals • 100% whole-grain mini bagels • 8-oz. servings of low-fat, fruit-flavored yogurt with ≤30 g of total sugars • Low-sodium, whole-grain bars containing sunflower seeds, almonds, or walnuts† • 8-oz. servings of low-fat or nonfat chocolate or strawberry milk with ≤22 g of total sugars † *The fat content of nuts and seeds does not count against the total fat content of combination **products**.*

3 = Yes, **all** competitive foods align with the IOM criteria, **or** we do not offer competitive foods at our school.
2 = **Most** competitive foods align with the IOM criteria.
1 = **Some** competitive foods align with the IOM criteria.
0 = No, **no** competitive foods align with the IOM criteria.

N.4 All beverages offered or sold during the school day meet strong nutrition standards

Do all beverages offered or sold during the school day outside the federal meal program align with the criteria recommended by the Institute of Medicine's Nutrition Standards for Foods in Schools (see criteria below)?

Nutrition Standards for Foods in Schools (Elementary) for Question N.4
BEVERAGES ARE LIMITED TO • Water (unflavored, non-carbonated) • Low-fat or nonfat milk in 8 oz. portions (includes lactose-free milk and soy beverages) • Low-fat or nonfat flavored milk with no more than 22 g total sugars per 8 oz. portion • 100-percent fruit juice (4 oz. portion in elementary school)

3 = Yes, **all** beverages offered or sold align with the IOM criteria, **or** we do not offer competitive foods at our school.

2 = **Most** beverages align with the IOM criteria.

1 = **Some** beverages align with the IOM criteria.

0 = No, **no** beverages offered or sold outside the federal meal program align with the IOM criteria.

N.5 Fundraising efforts during and outside school hours meet strong nutrition standards

Do fundraising efforts during and **outside school hours** sell only non-food items or foods and beverages that align with the criteria recommended by the Institute of Medicine's Nutrition Standards for Foods in Schools (see criteria below)?

Nutrition Standards for Foods in Schools for Question N.5	
Criteria for During and Outside School Hours	Examples
FOODS/SNACKS ARE LIMITED TO • Fruits or vegetables (e.g., fresh, canned, dried) • Whole grain snacks • Combination snacks (e.g., made of fruit and whole grain) • Nonfat and <u>low-fat</u> dairy products FOODS/SNACKS MUST ALSO BE • ≤200 calories • ≤35% total calories from fat • <10% of calories from saturated fats • Trans fat-free • ≤35% calories from total sugars • ≤200 mg of sodium ENTREE ITEMS ARE • National School Lunch Program (NSLP) menu items • ≤35% total calories from fat • <10% of calories from saturated fats • Trans fat-free • ≤35% calories from total sugars • Have a sodium content of 480 mg or less BEVERAGES ARE LIMITED TO • Water (unflavored, non-carbonated) • Low-fat or nonfat milk in 8 oz. portions (includes lactose-free milk and soy beverages) • Low-fat or nonfat flavored milk with no more than 22 g total sugars per 8 oz. portion • 100% fruit juice (4 oz. portion in elementary school)	• Individual fruits (apples, pears, oranges) • Fruit cups packed in juice or water • Vegetables (baby carrots, broccoli, edamame) • Dried or dehydrated fruits (raisins, apricots, cherries) • 100% fruit juice or low-sodium 100% vegetable juice • Low-fat, low-salt, whole-grain crackers or chips • Whole-grain, low-sugar cereals • 100% whole-grain mini bagels • 8-oz. servings of low-fat, fruit-flavored yogurt with ≤30 g of total sugars • Low-sodium, whole-grain bars containing sunflower seeds, almonds, or walnuts† • 8-oz. servings of low-fat or nonfat chocolate or strawberry milk with ≤22 g of total sugars † *The fat content of nuts and seeds does not count against the total fat content of combination products.*

3 = Yes, fundraising efforts only sell non-food items, or **all** food and beverage items sold as fundraisers align with these standards.
2 = **Most** food and beverage items sold as fundraisers align with these standards.
1 = **Some** food and beverage items sold as fundraisers align with these standards.
0 = No, the food and beverage items sold as fundraisers do **not** align with these standards.

N.6 Advertising and promotion of foods and beverages

Does your school limit food and beverage advertising and promotion (e.g., contests or coupons) on school property to foods and beverages that align with the criteria recommended by the Institute of Medicine's Nutrition Standards for Foods in Schools (see criteria in N.7)?

3= Yes, **only** foods and beverages that align with the IOM criteria are advertised or promoted, **or** no foods and beverages are advertised or promoted on school property.
2= **Most** foods and beverages advertised or promoted on school property align with the IOM criteria.
1= **Some** foods and beverages advertised or promoted on school property align with the IOM criteria.
0= No, **no** foods and beverages advertised or promoted on school property align with the IOM criteria.

N.7   Hands washed before meals and snacks

Do all teachers schedule time for students to wash their hands before meals and snacks?

3 = Yes, **all** do.
2 = **Most** do.
1 = **Some** do.
0 = **None** do.

T.1   Prohibit tobacco use among students

Does your school prohibit the **use of tobacco** by students, 24 hours a day, 7 days a week in the following locations?
- ✓ In all school buildings (including during extracurricular events)
- ✓ On all school grounds (including during extracurricular events)
- ✓ At all school-sponsored events off school grounds
- ✓ In all school vehicles

3 = Yes, in all locations.
2 = Tobacco use by students is prohibited in all school buildings and on all school grounds, but is allowed **either** at school-sponsored events off school grounds **or** in school vehicles.
1 = Tobacco use by students is prohibited only in school buildings, but is allowed on school grounds **or** tobacco use is allowed at **both** school-sponsored events off school grounds **and** in school vehicles.
0 = Tobacco use by students is allowed in school buildings **or** tobacco use is allowed on school grounds, at school-sponsored events off school grounds, **and** in school vehicles.

T.2   Prohibit tobacco use among school staff members and visitors

Does your school prohibit the **use of tobacco** by **staff members** and visitors, 24 hours a day, 7 days a week in the following locations?
- ✓ In all school buildings (including during extracurricular events)
- ✓ On all school grounds (including during extracurricular events)
- ✓ At all school-sponsored events off school grounds
- ✓ In all school vehicles

3 = Yes, in all locations.
2 = Tobacco use by staff members and visitors is prohibited in all school buildings and on all school grounds, but is allowed **either** at school-sponsored events off school grounds **or** in school vehicles.
1 = Tobacco use by staff members and visitors is prohibited only in school buildings, but is allowed on school grounds **or** tobacco use is allowed at **both** school-sponsored events off school grounds **and** in school vehicles.
0 = Tobacco use by staff members and visitors is allowed in school buildings **or** tobacco use is allowed on school grounds, at school-sponsored events off school grounds, **and** in school vehicles.

T.3 Enforce tobacco-use policies

Does your school handle violations of the tobacco-use **policies** in each of the following ways?
- ✓ Designating individual(s) to enforce the policy
- ✓ Having written policies for addressing violations by students, staff, and visitors
- ✓ Providing educational opportunities (e.g., tobacco-use prevention education sessions, tobacco cessation sessions) and not using solely punitive measures (e.g., detention, suspension)
- ✓ Referring students to the school counselor or nurse
- ✓ Tracking the frequency of violations by students so that repeat offenders can be identified and receive heavier consequences and more intense prevention or cessation assistance and/or referrals.
- ✓ Communicating violations to parents

3 = Yes, in each of these **six** ways.
2 = In **four or five** of these ways.
1 = In **one to three** of these ways.
0 = In **none** of these ways.

T.4 Prohibit tobacco advertising

Does your school prohibit advertising and displaying of tobacco-industry brand names, logos, and other identifiers in each of the following locations?
- ✓ On school property
- ✓ At other places where school functions occur
- ✓ In school-developed or school-sponsored publications
- ✓ On students' and **staff members**' clothing, shoes, and accessories
- ✓ On students' and staff members' gear and school supplies (e.g., backpacks, lunchboxes, games, book covers, other personal items)

3 = Yes, in each of these **five** locations.
2 = In **three or four** of these locations.
1 = In **one or two** of these locations.
0 = In **none** of these locations.

A.1 Written policies for carry and self-administration of quick-relief medications

Does your school or district have written **policies** that permit students to carry and self-administer prescribed quick-relief medications for asthma that include all of the following?
- ✓ Approval from authorized prescriber (e.g., MD, DO, PNP, etc.)
- ✓ Approval from parent/guardian
- ✓ Approval from school nurse
- ✓ Request for back-up medication to be kept in the school health office
- ✓ Student contract with clear rules and consequences for violations
- ✓ Immediate notification of parent/guardian if permission is withdrawn
- ✓ Annual parental notification about policy

3 = Yes, our school has written policies that include **all** of these components.
2 = Our school has written policies that include **most** of these components.
1 = Our school has written policies that include **only a few** of these components.
0 = No, our school does **not** have written policies, **or** the policies do not include any of these components.

A.2 Professional development on asthma

Have all **staff members** received **professional development** on **asthma basics and emergency response** in the past two years?

3 = Yes, **all** staff members have received professional development on asthma management.
2 = **Most** staff members have received professional development on asthma management.
1 = **Some** staff members have received professional development on asthma management.
0 = **No** staff members have received professional development on asthma management.

A.3 Implement indoor air quality practices

Does your school consistently implement all of the following indoor air quality practices?

✓ Regularly clean and vacuum when students are not in school (consider using vacuums with high efficiency particulate filters (HEPA) or central vacuums where carpeting exists)

✓ Respond quickly to signs of moisture, including mold, mildew, and water leaks in the building (e.g., plumbing) and around the building envelope (e.g., doors, windows, roof)

✓ Prevent exhaust fumes from entering the school or accumulating in the outdoor areas by prohibiting buses and cars from idling outside of the school building

✓ Maintain adequate ventilation throughout the building

✓ Schedule regular maintenance and repair for heating, ventilation, and air condition (HVAC) system

✓ Reduce or eliminate exposure to furred and feathered animals

✓ Schedule painting and major building maintenance or renovations during times when school is not in session, and isolate renovation areas so that dust and debris are confined

3 = Yes, **all** of these practices are implemented consistently.
2 = **Most** of these practices are implemented consistently.
1 = **Only a few** of these practices are implemented consistently.
0 = **None** of these practices are implemented consistently.

A.4 Implement integrated pest management practices

Does your school consistently use the safest and lowest risk approach to controlling problems with **pests** by implementing the following integrated pest management practices?

✓ Monitor potential pest infestations with regular and careful inspections

✓ Use adequate sanitation practices (e.g., cover trash cans, place dumpsters away from buildings) and structural modifications (caulking & screening) to minimize pests

✓ Use proper food handling, preparation, and storage techniques

✓ Use non-chemical pest management techniques, such as sticky traps, pheromone traps, and insect light traps prior to using chemical-based techniques

✓ Use pesticides or herbicides as a last resort method when no alternative measures are practical and when students and **staff members** are not in the area; refrain from regular pesticide application

✓ Notify parents, employees, and students of all pesticide and herbicide use

3 = Yes, **all** of these practices are implemented consistently.
2 = **Most** of these practices are implemented consistently.
1 = **Only a few** of these practices are implemented consistently.
0 = **None** of these practices are implemented consistently.

SH.1 Non-discrimination on the basis of HIV infection policy

Does your school implement a non-discrimination policy, within the context of federal, state, or local requirements, that protects HIV infected students and **staff members** and includes all of the following components?

✓ Children with HIV/AIDS can attend school in regular classrooms without restrictions by reason of HIV alone
✓ Known HIV positive students are allowed to fully participate in **physical education**, **recess**, competitive sports, extracurricular school-sponsored activities, and other physical activity programs
✓ **Harassment** or **bullying** of HIV infected students and staff members is not tolerated
✓ Reasonable accommodation is made for necessary school absences (e.g., medically-necessary absences are excused, re-enrollment procedures are straightforward and not time-consuming)
✓ Procedural safeguards are in place for **corrective action** when discrimination is alleged to have occurred (e.g., an impartial hearing with an opportunity for participation by the parents or guardians and representation by counsel, a review procedure)

3 = Yes, our school implements a non-discrimination policy that includes all **five** of these components.
2 = Our school implements a non-discrimination policy that includes **four** of these components.
1 = Our school implements a non-discrimination policy that includes **one to three** of these components.
0 = Our school's non-discrimination policy does **not** include any of these components, **or** we do not have such a non-discrimination policy.

SH.2 Confidentiality of HIV status

Does your school implement a confidentiality of HIV status policy, within the context of federal, state, or local requirements that includes all of the following components?

✓ Students or **staff members** are not required to disclose HIV status to anyone
✓ HIV antibody testing is not required for any purpose
✓ HIV status will not be divulged without court order or informed, written, signed, and dated consent of the person with HIV infection (or parent/guardian of legal minor) in compliance with federal, state or local requirements
✓ Health records, notes, and other documents that reference HIV status will be kept under lock and key
✓ Access to confidential records is limited to those named in written permission from the person (or parent/guardian) and to emergency medical personnel
✓ Information regarding HIV status will not be added to student's permanent educational or health record without written consent from the student (or parent/guardian of legal minor)
✓ Procedural safeguards for **corrective action** for policy violation

3 = Yes, our school implements a confidentiality of HIV status policy that includes all **seven** of these components.
2 = Our school implements a confidentiality of HIV status policy that includes **six** of these components.
1 = Our school implements a confidentiality of HIV status policy that includes **one to five** of these components.
0 = Our school's confidentiality of HIV status policy does **not** include any of these components, **or** we do not have a confidentiality of HIV status policy.

SH.3 Professional development for all staff members on HIV policies or laws

Have all **staff members** received **professional development** on the following HIV **policies** or laws, and enforcement of policies or laws, in the past two years?
✓ Attendance of students with HIV infection in regular classrooms without restrictions
✓ Procedures to protect HIV-infected students and staff members from discrimination
✓ Maintaining confidentiality of HIV-infected students and staff members

3 = Yes, **all** staff members have received professional development on HIV policies or laws.
2 = **Most** staff members have received professional development on HIV policies or laws.
1 = **Some** staff members have received professional development on HIV policies or laws.
0 = **No** staff members have received professional development on HIV policies or laws **or** staff members have not received this professional development in the past two years.

SH.4 Professional development for administrators and teachers on HIV, other STD, and pregnancy prevention

Have administrators and teachers received **professional development** on **HIV, other STD, and pregnancy prevention** in the past two years?

3 = Yes, **all** administrators and teachers have received professional development on HIV, other STD, and pregnancy prevention.

2 = **Most** administrators and teachers have received professional development on HIV, other STD, and pregnancy prevention.

1 = **Some** administrators and teachers have received professional development on HIV, other STD, and pregnancy prevention.

0 = **No** administrators and teachers have received professional development on HIV, other STD, and pregnancy prevention, **or** staff members have not received this professional development in the past two years.

This page intentionally left blank.

Module 1: School Health and Safety Policies and Environment

Planning Questions
(photocopy before using)

The Module 1 Planning Questions will help your school use its School Health Index results to identify and prioritize changes that will improve policies and programs to improve students' health and safety.

Planning Question 1
Look back at the scores you assigned to each question. According to these scores, what are the **strengths** and the **weaknesses** of your school's policies and environment related to students' health and safety?

Planning Question 2
For each of the weaknesses identified above, list several recommended actions to improve the school's scores (e.g., create and maintain a school health committee).

Continued on next page

SCHOOL HEALTH INDEX – ELEMENTARY SCHOOL

Planning Question 3. List each of the actions identified in Planning Question 2 on the table below. Use the five-point scales defined below to rank each action on five dimensions (importance, cost, time, commitment, feasibility). Add the points for each action to get the total points. Use the total points to help you choose one, two, or three top priority actions that you will recommend to the School Health Index team for implementation this year.

Importance	**How important is the action to my school?**		
	5 = Very important	3 = Moderately important	1 = Not important
Cost	**How expensive would it be to plan and implement the action?**		
	5 = Not expensive	3 = Moderately expensive	1 = Very expensive
Time	**How much time and effort would it take to implement the action?**		
	5 = Little or no time and effort	3 = Moderate time and effort	1 = Very great time and effort
Commitment	**How enthusiastic would the school community be about implementing the action?**		
	5 = Very enthusiastic	3 = Moderately enthusiastic	1 = Not enthusiastic
Feasibility	**How difficult would it be to complete the action?**		
	5 = Not difficult	3 = Moderately difficult	1 = Very difficult

Module 1 Actions	Importance	Cost	Time	Commitment	Feasibility	Total Points	Top Priority Action?

Module 2: Health Education

Instructions for Module Coordinator

Habits and practices related to health and safety are influenced by the entire school environment. That's why the School Health Index has eight different modules, which correspond to the eight components of coordinated school health in the figure below.

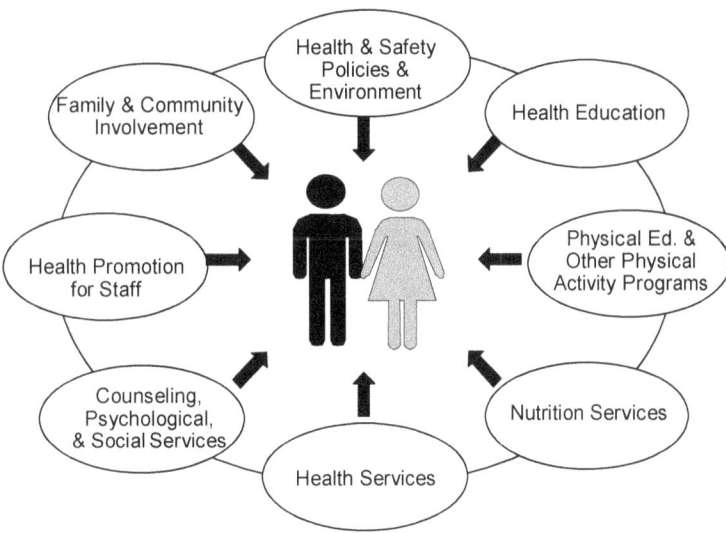

Instructions for completing the module

1. Work with the site coordinator to organize a team to complete the module's documents. Below are some suggested members for the Module 2 team.

Health education teacher(s)	Parent(s)
Physical education teacher(s)	Student(s)
Other teacher(s)	School counselor
School nutrition services manager	School custodial staff
School nurse	Health department representative
School security personnel	Assistant principal

2. Make a photocopy of the module Discussion Questions (pages 5-15) for each Module 2 team member. Make at least one photocopy of the module Score Card (page 3) and the module Planning Questions (pages 17-18).

3. Give each Module 2 team member a copy of the Module 2 Discussion Questions. Use the copies of the module Score Card and the Planning Questions to record the team's work. Put the originals of these documents away in case you need to make more photocopies.

4. At a Module 2 team meeting:
   - Discuss each of the Module 2 Discussion Questions and its scoring choices.
   - Decide how to collect any information you need to answer each question accurately.
   - After you have all the information you need, arrive at a consensus score for each question. Answer each question as accurately as possible. The School Health Index is **your** self-assessment tool for identifying strengths and weaknesses and for planning improvements; it should not be used for evaluating staff.
   - Record the scores (0 to 3) for each question on the module Score Card and calculate the overall Module Score.
   - Use the scores written on the module Score Card to complete the Planning Questions at the end of the module.
   - Use the results from the third Planning Question to identify the one, two, or three highest priority actions that you will recommend to the School Health Index team for implementation this year.
   - Use the answers to the Planning Questions to decide how you will present your results and recommendations at the follow-up School Health Index team meeting.

We wish you success in your efforts to improve the health and safety of young people!

Module 2: Health Education

Score Card
(photocopy before using)

Instructions
1. Carefully read and discuss the Module 2 Discussion Questions (pages 5-15), which contains questions and scoring descriptions for each item listed on this Score Card.
2. Circle the most appropriate score for each item.
3. After all questions have been scored, calculate the overall Module Score and complete the Module 2 Planning Questions located at the end of this module (pages 17-18).

		Fully in Place	Partially in Place	Under Develop-ment	Not in Place
CC.1	Health education taught in all grades	3	2	1	0
CC.2	Sequential health education curriculum consistent with standards	3	2	1	0
CC.3	Active learning strategies	3	2	1	0
CC.4	Opportunities to practice skills	3	2	1	0
CC.5	Culturally appropriate activities and examples	3	2	1	0
CC.6	Assignments encourage student interaction with family and community	3	2	1	0
CC.7	Professional development in health education	3	2	1	0
CC.8	Professional development in delivering curriculum	3	2	1	0
CC.9	Professional development in classroom management techniques	3	2	1	0
S.1	Essential topics on preventing unintentional injuries, violence, and suicide	3	2	1	0
PA.1	Essential topics on physical activity	3	2	1	0
N.1	Essential topics on healthy eating	3	2	1	0
T.1	Essential topics on preventing tobacco use	3	2	1	0
A.1	Essential topics on asthma awareness	3	2	1	0
SH.1	Essential topics for preventing HIV, other STD and pregnancy	3	2	1	0

COLUMN TOTALS: For each column, add up the numbers that are circled and enter the sum in this row.

(If you decide to skip any of the topic areas, make sure you adjust the denominator for the Module Score (45) by subtracting 3 for each question eliminated).

TOTAL POINTS: Add the four sums above and enter the total to the right.

MODULE SCORE =
(Total Points / 45) X 100

%

This page intentionally left blank.

Module 2: Health Education

Discussion Questions

CC.1   Health education taught in all grades

Do students receive health education instruction in all grades?

3 = Yes, in <u>all</u> grades.
2 = In <u>most</u> grades.
1 = In <u>some</u> grades.
0 = In <u>no</u> grades.

CC.2 Sequential health education curriculum consistent with standards

Do all teachers of health education use an age-appropriate **sequential** health education curriculum that is **consistent** with state or national standards for health education (see standards box)?

NOTE: Consider using CDC's *Health Education Curriculum Analysis Tool* (HECAT), which is designed to help school districts and schools conduct a clear, complete, and consistent analysis of written health education curriculum. HECAT results can help districts and schools enhance, develop, or select appropriate and effective health education curricula. The HECAT assesses how consistent curricula are with national standards and can assist users in determining if the curriculum being analyzed is sequential.

3 = Yes.
2 = **Some** teachers use a sequential health education curriculum, **and** it is consistent with state or national standards.
1 = **Some** teachers use a sequential health education curriculum, **but** it is not consistent with state or national standards.
0 = None do, **or** the curriculum is not sequential, **or** there is no health education curriculum.

National Health Education Standards
(For Question CC.2)

1. Students will comprehend concepts related to health promotion and disease prevention to enhance health.
2. Students will analyze the influence of family, peers, culture, media, technology, and other factors on health behaviors.
3. Students will demonstrate the ability to access valid information and products and services to enhance health.
4. Students will demonstrate the ability to use interpersonal communication skills to enhance health and avoid or reduce health risks.
5. Students will demonstrate the ability to use decision-making skills to enhance health.
6. Students will demonstrate the ability to use goal-setting skills to enhance health.
7. Students will demonstrate the ability to practice health-enhancing behaviors and avoid or reduce health risks.
8. Students will demonstrate the ability to advocate for personal, family, and community health.

Joint Committee on National Health Education Standards. *National health education standards: achieving excellence*, 2nd edition. 2007.

CC.3   Active learning strategies

Do all teachers of health education use **active learning strategies** and activities that students find enjoyable and personally relevant?

3 = Yes, **all** do.
2 = **Most** do.
1 = **Some** do.
0 = **None** do, **or** no one teaches health education.

CC.4   Opportunities to practice skills

Do all teachers of health education provide opportunities for students to practice or rehearse the **skills needed to maintain and improve their health**?

3 = Yes, **all** do.
2 = **Most** do.
1 = **Some** do.
0 = **None** do, **or** no one teaches health education.

CC.5   Culturally-appropriate activities and examples

Do all teachers of health education use a variety of **culturally-appropriate activities and examples** that reflect the community's cultural diversity?

3 = Yes, **all** do.
2 = **Most** do.
1 = **Some** do.
0 = **None** do, **or** no one teaches health education.

CC.6   Assignments encourage student interaction with family and community

Do all teachers of health education use assignments or projects that encourage students to have **interactions with family members and community organizations**?

3 = Yes, **all** do.
2 = **Most** do.
1 = **Some** do.
0 = **None** do, **or** no one teaches health education.

CC.7 Professional development in health education

Do all teachers of health education participate at least once a year in **professional development** in health education?

3 = Yes, **all** do.
2 = **Most** do.
1 = **Some** do.
0 = **None** do, **or** no one teaches health education.

CC.8 Professional development in delivering curriculum

Have all teachers of health education received **professional development** in **delivery** of the school's health and safety curriculum in the past two years?

3 = Yes, **all** have.
2 = **Most** have.
1 = **Some** have.
0 = **None** have.

CC.9 Professional development in classroom management techniques

Have all teachers received **professional development** in **classroom management techniques** in the past two years?

3 = Yes, **all** have.
2 = **Most** have.
1 = **Some** have.
0 = **None** have.

S.1 Essential topics to prevent unintentional injuries and violence

Does your health education curriculum address all of these topics on preventing unintentional injuries and violence?

Unintentional injury-related topics include:
- ✓ Motor vehicle occupant safety, such as seatbelt use
- ✓ Fire, water, pedestrian and playground safety
- ✓ Poisoning prevention
- ✓ Use of protective equipment for biking, skating or other sports
- ✓ First aid and cardiopulmonary resuscitation (CPR)
- ✓ Emergency preparedness

Violence-related topics include:
- ✓ Anger management
- ✓ **Bullying** and what to do if someone is being bullied
- ✓ Teasing
- ✓ Personal safety, for example, dealing with strangers
- ✓ Inappropriate touching
- ✓ Techniques to resolve conflicts without fighting
- ✓ Prosocial behaviors, such as cooperation, praise, or showing support for others
- ✓ Recognize signs and symptoms of people who are in danger of hurting themselves or others
- ✓ What to do if someone is thinking about hurting himself or herself or others
- ✓ Short- and long-term consequences of violence
- ✓ Relationship between suicide and other types of violence and between suicide and emotional and mental health
- ✓ When to seek help for suicidal thoughts

General injury-related topics include:
- ✓ Prejudice, discrimination, and bias
- ✓ Empathy, that is, identification with and understanding of another person's feelings, situation, or motives
- ✓ Perspective taking, that is, taking another person's point of view
- ✓ Relationship between alcohol or other drug use and injuries, violence and suicide
- ✓ Social influences on unintentional injury, violence and suicide, including media, family, peers, and culture
- ✓ How to find valid information or services to prevent injuries, violence and suicide
- ✓ How to resist peer pressure that would increase the risk of injuries, violence and suicide
- ✓ How to take steps to achieve the personal goal to prevent injuries, violence and suicide
- ✓ How to influence, support, or advocate for others to prevent injuries, violence and suicide

NOTE: Consider using CDC's *Health Education Curriculum Analysis Tool* (HECAT), which is designed to help school districts and schools conduct a clear, complete, and consistent analysis of written health education curriculum. HECAT results can help districts and schools enhance, develop, or select appropriate and effective health education curricula. The HECAT assesses how consistent curricula are with national standards and can assist users in determining if the curriculum being analyzed is sequential.

3 = Yes, addresses **all** of these topics.
2 = Addresses **most** of these topics.
1 = Addresses **some** of these topics.
0 = Addresses **one or none** of these topics, **or** there is no health education curriculum.

PA.1 Essential topics on physical activity

Does your health education curriculum address all of these topics on physical activity?
- ✓ The physical, psychological, or social benefits of physical activity
- ✓ How physical activity can contribute to a healthy weight
- ✓ How physical activity can contribute to the academic learning process
- ✓ How an inactive lifestyle contributes to chronic disease
- ✓ Health-related fitness, that is, cardiovascular endurance, muscular endurance, muscular strength, flexibility, and body composition
- ✓ Differences between physical activity, exercise, and fitness
- ✓ Phases of an exercise session, that is, warm up, workout, and cool down
- ✓ Overcoming barriers to physical activity
- ✓ Decreasing sedentary activities, such as TV watching
- ✓ Opportunities for physical activity in the community
- ✓ Preventing injury during physical activity
- ✓ Weather-related safety, for example, avoiding heat stroke, hypothermia, and sunburn while physically active
- ✓ Social influences on physical activity, including media, family, peers, and culture
- ✓ How to find valid information or services related to physical activity and fitness
- ✓ How to take steps to achieve the personal goal to be physically active
- ✓ How to influence, support, or advocate for others to engage in physical activity
- ✓ How to resist peer pressure that discourages physical activity

NOTE: Consider using CDC's *Health Education Curriculum Analysis Tool* (HECAT), which is designed to help school districts and schools conduct a clear, complete, and consistent analysis of written health education curriculum. HECAT results can help districts and schools enhance, develop, or select appropriate and effective health education curricula. The HECAT assesses how consistent curricula are with national standards and can assist users in determining if the curriculum being analyzed is sequential.

3 = Yes, addresses **all** of these topics.
2 = Addresses **most** of these topics.
1 = Addresses **some** of these topics.
0 = Addresses **one or none** of these topics, **or** there is no health education curriculum.

N.1 Essential topics on healthy eating

Does your health education curriculum address all of these essential topics on healthy eating?

✓ The relationship between healthy eating and personal health and disease prevention
✓ Food guidance from MyPlate or MyPyramid
✓ Reading and using food labels
✓ Eating a variety of foods every day
✓ Balancing food intake and physical activity
✓ Eating more fruits, vegetables and whole grain products
✓ Choosing foods that are low in fat, saturated fat, and cholesterol and do not contain transfat
✓ Choosing foods and beverages with little added sugars
✓ Eating more calcium-rich foods
✓ Preparing healthy meals and snacks
✓ Risks of unhealthy weight control practices
✓ Accepting body size differences
✓ Food safety
✓ Importance of water consumption
✓ Importance of eating breakfast
✓ Making healthy choices when eating at restaurants
✓ Social influences on healthy eating, including media, family, peers, and culture
✓ How to find valid information or services related to nutrition and dietary behavior
✓ How to take steps to achieve the personal goal to eat healthfully
✓ Resisting peer pressure related to unhealthy dietary behavior
✓ Influencing, supporting, or advocating for others' healthy dietary behavior

NOTE: Consider using CDC's *Health Education Curriculum Analysis Tool* (HECAT), which is designed to help school districts and schools conduct a clear, complete, and consistent analysis of written health education curriculum. HECAT results can help districts and schools enhance, develop, or select appropriate and effective health education curricula. The HECAT assesses how consistent curricula are with national standards and can assist users in determining if the curriculum being analyzed is sequential.

3 = Yes, addresses **all** of these topics.
2 = Addresses **most** of these topics.
1 = Addresses **some** of these topics.
0 = Addresses **one or none** of these topics, **or** there is no health education curriculum.

T.1 Essential topics on preventing tobacco use

Does your health education curriculum address all of these essential topics on preventing tobacco use?
- ✓ short- and long-term health consequences of tobacco use, including cigarettes, cigars and smokeless tobacco and other tobacco products
- ✓ benefits of abstaining from tobacco use
- ✓ importance of quitting tobacco use
- ✓ addictive effects of nicotine in tobacco products
- ✓ health effects of second-hand smoke and benefits of a smoke-free and overall tobacco-free environment
- ✓ how many young people use tobacco
- ✓ social influences on tobacco use, including media, family, peers, and culture
- ✓ finding valid information and services related to tobacco-use prevention and cessation
- ✓ resisting peer pressure to use tobacco
- ✓ making a personal commitment not to use tobacco
- ✓ supporting school and community action to support a tobacco-free environment
- ✓ influencing, supporting, or advocating for others to prevent tobacco use
- ✓ influencing or supporting others to quit using tobacco
- ✓ how to avoid environmental tobacco smoke or second-hand smoke

NOTE: Consider using CDC's *Health Education Curriculum Analysis Tool* (HECAT), which is designed to help school districts and schools conduct a clear, complete, and consistent analysis of written health education curriculum. HECAT results can help districts and schools enhance, develop, or select appropriate and effective health education curricula. The HECAT assesses how consistent curricula are with national standards and can assist users in determining if the curriculum being analyzed is sequential.

3 = Yes, addresses **all** of these topics.
2 = Addresses **most** of these topics.
1 = Addresses **some** of these topics.
0 = Addresses **one or none** of these topics, **or** there is no health education curriculum.

A.1 Essential topics on asthma awareness

Does your health education curriculum address all of these essential topics on asthma awareness?
- ✓ Basic facts and triggers of asthma
- ✓ Accessing a trusted adult who can help someone experiencing an asthma episode
- ✓ Ways to support classmates with asthma
- ✓ Demonstrating empathy for people with asthma

NOTE: Consider using CDC's *Health Education Curriculum Analysis Tool* (HECAT), which is designed to help school districts and schools conduct a clear, complete, and consistent analysis of written health education curriculum. HECAT results can help districts and schools enhance, develop, or select appropriate and effective health education curricula. The HECAT assesses how consistent curricula are with national standards and can assist users in determining if the curriculum being analyzed is sequential.

3 = Yes, addresses all **four** of these topics.
2 = Addresses **three** of these topics.
1 = Addresses **two** of these topics.
0 = Addresses **one or none** of these topics, **or** there is no health education curriculum.

SH.1 Essential topics to prevent HIV, other STD, and pregnancy

Does your health education curriculum address all of these essential topics to prevent HIV, other STD and pregnancy?

Early elementary school topics include:
- ✓ Establishing and maintaining healthy relationships
- ✓ Healthy ways to express affection, love, and friendship and to effectively communicate needs, wants, and feelings
- ✓ Why it is wrong to harass, tease, or bully others based on **gender identity** or **gender expression** and ways to show courtesy and respect for others whose gender identity or gender expression differ from one's own
- ✓ Ways that disease-causing germs are transmitted and how to prevent the spread of germs that cause common infectious diseases

Late elementary school topics include:
- ✓ Establishing and maintaining healthy relationships
- ✓ Healthy ways to express affection, love, and friendship and to effectively communicate needs, wants, and feelings
- ✓ Why it is wrong to harass, tease, or bully others based on gender identity or gender expression and ways to show courtesy and respect for others whose gender identity or gender expression differ from one's own
- ✓ Human development issues, including reproductive anatomy and puberty
- ✓ Ways that common infectious diseases are transmitted and ways to prevent the spread of germs that cause infectious diseases
- ✓ How HIV and other STD are transmitted and how they affect the human body
- ✓ Compassion for persons living with chronic diseases, including HIV or AIDS
- ✓ Social influences on risky behavior, including media, family, peers, **gender roles**, religious beliefs and culture
- ✓ Resisting peer pressure to engage in behaviors that increase risk for HIV, other STDs, and pregnancy.
- ✓ How to influence, support, or advocate for others to avoid engaging in behaviors that increase risk for HIV, other STDs, and pregnancy.

NOTE: Consider using CDC's *Health Education Curriculum Analysis Tool* (HECAT), which is designed to help school districts and schools conduct a clear, complete, and consistent analysis of written health education curriculum. HECAT results can help districts and schools enhance, develop, or select appropriate and effective health education curricula. The HECAT assesses how consistent curricula are with national standards and can assist users in determining if the curriculum being analyzed is sequential.

3 = Yes, addresses **all** of these topics.
2 = Addresses **most** of these topics.
1 = Addresses **some** of these topics.
0 = Addresses **one or none** of these topics, **or** there is no health education curriculum.

This page intentionally left blank.

Module 2: Health Education

Planning Questions
(photocopy before using)

The Module 2 Planning Questions will help your school use its School Health Index results to identify and prioritize changes that will improve policies and programs to improve students' health and safety.

Planning Question 1
Look back at the scores you assigned to each question. According to these scores, what are the **strengths** and the **weaknesses** of your school's health education program related to students' health and safety?

Planning Question 2
For each of the weaknesses identified above, list several recommended actions to improve the school's scores (e.g., require students to receive health education instruction in all grades).

Continued on next page

Planning Question 3. List each of the actions identified in Planning Question 2 on the table below. Use the five-point scales defined below to rank each action on five dimensions (importance, cost, time, commitment, feasibility). Add the points for each action to get the total points. Use the total points to help you choose one, two, or three top priority actions that you will recommend to the School Health Index team for implementation this year.

Importance	How important is the action to my school?		
	5 = Very important	3 = Moderately important	1 = Not important
Cost	How expensive would it be to plan and implement the action?		
	5 = Not expensive	3 = Moderately expensive	1 = Very expensive
Time	How much time and effort would it take to implement the action?		
	5 = Little or no time and effort	3 = Moderate time and effort	1 = Very great time and effort
Commitment	How enthusiastic would the school community be about implementing the action?		
	5 = Very enthusiastic	3 = Moderately enthusiastic	1 = Not enthusiastic
Feasibility	How difficult would it be to complete the action?		
	5 = Not difficult	3 = Moderately difficult	1 = Very difficult

Module 2 Actions	Importance	Cost	Time	Commitment	Feasibility	Total Points	Top Priority Action?

Module 3: Physical Education and Other Physical Activity Programs

Instructions for Module Coordinator

Habits and practices related to health and safety are influenced by the entire school environment. That's why the School Health Index has eight different modules, which correspond to the eight components of coordinated school health in the figure below.

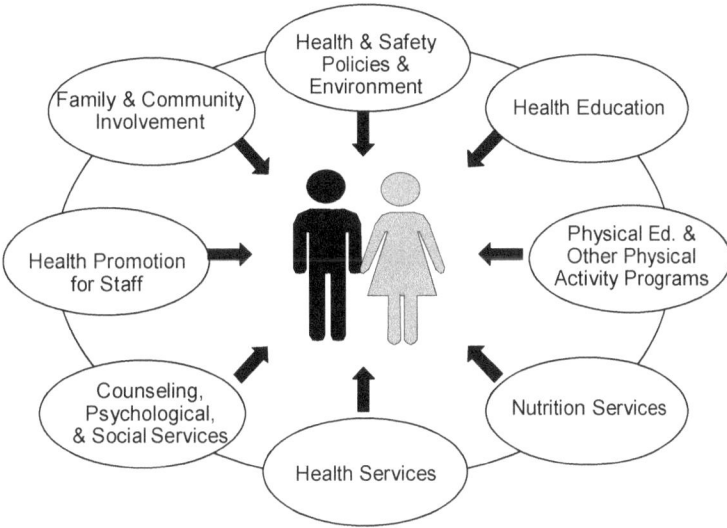

Instructions for completing the module

1. Work with the site coordinator to organize a team to complete the module's documents. Below are some suggested members of the Module 3 team.

Physical education teacher	Parent(s)
Teacher(s)	Student(s)
Athletic coach(es)	Community member(s)
School nurse	Assistant principal

2. Make a photocopy of the module Discussion Questions (pages 5-14) for each Module 3 team member. Make at least one photocopy of the module Score Card (page 3) and the module Planning Questions (pages 15-16).

3. Give each Module 3 team member a copy of the Module 3 Discussion Questions. Use the copies of the module Score Card and the Planning Questions to record the team's work. Put the originals of these documents away in case you need to make more photocopies.

4. At a Module 3 team meeting:
   - Discuss each of the Module 3 Discussion Questions and its scoring choices.
   - Decide how to collect any information you need to answer each question accurately.
   - After you have all the information you need, arrive at a consensus score for each question. Answer each question as accurately as possible. The School Health Index is **your** self-assessment tool for identifying strengths and weaknesses and for planning improvements; it should not be used for evaluating staff.
   - Record the scores (0-3) for each question on the module Score Card and calculate the overall Module Score.
   - Use the scores written on the module Score Card to complete the Planning Questions at the end of the module.
   - Use the results from the third Planning Question to identify the one, two, or three highest priority actions that you will recommend to the School Health Index team for implementation this year.
   - Use the answers to the Planning Questions to decide how you will present your results and recommendations at the follow-up School Health Index team meeting.

We wish you success in your efforts to improve the health and safety of young people!

Module 3: Physical Education and Other Physical Activity Programs

Score Card
(photocopy before using)

Instructions
1. Carefully read and discuss the Module 3 Discussion Questions (pages 5-14), which contains questions and scoring descriptions for each item listed on this Score Card.
2. Circle the most appropriate score for each item.
3. After all questions have been scored, calculate the overall Module Score and complete the Module 3 Planning Questions located at the end of this module (pages 15-16).

		Fully in Place	Partially in Place	Under Develop-ment	Not in Place
PA.1	150 minutes of physical education per week	3	2	1	0
PA.2	Adequate teacher/student ratio	3	2	1	0
PA.3	Sequential physical education curriculum consistent with standards	3	2	1	0
PA.4	Information and materials for physical education teachers	3	2	1	0
PA.5	Prohibit exemptions or waivers for physical education	3	2	1	0
PA.6	Students active at least 50% of class time	3	2	1	0
PA.7	Individualized physical activity and fitness plans	3	2	1	0
PA.8	Health-related fitness	3	2	1	0
PA.9	Teachers avoid practices that result in student inactivity				
PA.10	Promote community physical activities	3	2	1	0
PA.11	Certified or licensed physical education teachers	3	2	1	0
PA.12/A.1	Address special health care needs	3	2	1	0
PA.13/ S.1/A.2	Physical education safety practices	3	2	1	0
PA.14/S.2	Playgrounds meet safety standards	3	2	1	0
PA.15	Professional development for teachers	3	2	1	0
PA.16	Participation in intramural programs or physical activity clubs	3	2	1	0
PA.17	Promotion or support of walking and bicycling to school	3	2	1	0
PA.18/S.3	Physical activity facilities meet safety standards	3	2	1	0

COLUMN TOTALS: For each column, add up the numbers that are circled and enter the sum in this row.

(If you decide to skip any of the topic areas, make sure you adjust the denominator for the Module Score (54) by subtracting 3 for each question eliminated).

TOTAL POINTS: Add the four sums above and enter the total to the right.

MODULE SCORE =
(Total Points / 54) X 100   %

This page intentionally left blank.

Module 3: Physical Education and Other Physical Activity Programs

Discussion Questions

PA.1   150 minutes of physical education per week

Do all students in each grade receive **physical education** for at least 150 minutes per week throughout the school year?

NOTE: Physical education classes should be spread over at least three days per week, with daily physical education preferable.

3 = Yes.
2 = **90-149 minutes** per week for all students in each grade throughout the school year.
1 = **60-89 minutes** per week for all students in each grade throughout the school year.
0 = **Fewer than 60** minutes per week **or** not all students receive physical education throughout the school year.

PA.2   Adequate teacher/student ratio

Do **physical education** classes have a student/teacher ratio **comparable** to that of other classes?

NOTE: Aides and volunteers should not be counted as teachers in the student/teacher ratio.

3 = Yes.
2 = The ratio is **somewhat** larger (up to one and a half times larger) than the ratio for most other classes.
1 = The ratio is **considerably** larger (more than one and a half times larger), **but** there are plans to reduce it.
0 = The ratio is **considerably** larger (more than one and a half times larger), **and** there are no plans to reduce it.

PA.3   Sequential physical education curriculum consistent with standards

Do all teachers of **physical education** use an age-appropriate, **sequential** physical education curriculum that is **consistent** with national or state standards for physical education (see national standards below)?

NOTE: Consider using CDC's *Physical Education Curriculum Analysis Tool* (PECAT), which is designed to help school districts and schools conduct a clear, complete, and consistent analysis of written physical education curriculum. PECAT results can help districts and schools enhance, develop, or select appropriate and effective physical education curricula for delivering high-quality physical education in schools. The PECAT assesses how consistent curricula are with national standards and can assist users in determining if the curriculum being analyzed is sequential.

3 = Yes.
2 = **Some** use a sequential physical education curriculum, **and** it is consistent with state or national standards.
1 = **Some** use a sequential physical education curriculum, **but** it is not consistent with state or national standards.
0 = **None** do, **or** the curriculum is not sequential, **or** there is no physical education curriculum.

National Standards for Physical Education
(For Question PA.3)

A physically educated person:
1. Demonstrates competency in motor skills and movement patterns needed to perform a variety of physical activities.
2. Demonstrates understanding of movement concepts, principles, strategies, and tactics as they apply to the learning and performance of physical activities.
3. Participates regularly in physical activity.
4. Achieves and maintains a health-enhancing level of physical fitness.
5. Exhibits responsible personal and social behavior that respects self and others in physical activity settings.
6. Values physical activity for health, enjoyment, challenge, self-expression, and/or social interaction.

National Association for Sport and Physical Education. *Moving into the Future: National Standards for Physical Education.* 2nd ed. Reston, VA: National Association for Sport and Physical Education, 2004.

PA.4 Information and materials for physical education teachers

Are all teachers of **physical education** provided with the following information and materials to assist in delivering quality physical education?
✓ Goals, objectives, and expected outcomes for physical education
✓ A written physical education curriculum
✓ A chart scope and sequence for instruction
✓ A plan for assessing student performance

3 = Yes, all teachers of physical education are provided with all **four** kinds of materials.
2 = Teachers of physical education are provided with **three** kinds of these materials.
1 = Teachers of physical education are provided with **one or two** kinds of these materials.
0 = Teachers of physical education are **not** provided with these kinds of materials.

PA.5   Prohibit exemptions or waivers for physical education

Does the school **prohibit exemptions or waivers** for **physical education**?

3 = Yes.
2 = Yes, **bu**t occasional exceptions or waivers are made.
1 = No, **but** there are plans to start prohibiting exemptions or waivers.
0 = No, **or** there is no physical education.

PA.6   Students active at least 50% of class time

Do teachers keep students **moderately to vigorously active** for **at least 50% of the time** during most or all **physical education** class sessions?

3 = Yes, during **most or all** classes.
2 = During **about half** the classes.
1 = During **fewer than half** the classes.
0 = During **none** of the classes, **or** there are no physical education classes.

PA.7   Individualized physical activity and fitness plans

Do students design and implement their own **individualized physical activity and fitness plans** as part of the **physical education** program? Do teachers of physical education provide ongoing feedback to students on progress in implementing their plans?

3 = Yes.
2 = Students design and implement their own individualized plans, **but** teachers provide only occasional feedback.
1 = Students design and implement their own individualized plans, **but** teachers provide no feedback.
0 = Students do not design and implement their own individualized plans, **or** there is no physical education program.

PA.8 Health-related physical fitness

Does the **physical education** program **integrate instruction** on **health-related fitness** into most lessons throughout the year?

3 = Yes, into **most** lessons.
2 = Into **about half** the lessons.
1 = Into **fewer than half** the lessons.
0 = Into **none** of the lessons, **or** there is no physical education program.

PA.9   Teachers avoid practices that result in student inactivity

Do teachers avoid using **practices** that result in some students spending considerable time being inactive in **physical education** classes?

3 = They **never** use such practices.
2 = They **rarely** use such practices.
1 = They **occasionally** use such practices.
0 = They **frequently** use such practices, **or** there are no physical education classes.

PA.10 Promote community physical activities

Does the **physical education** program use three or more **methods to promote student participation** in a variety of **community physical activity options**?

3 = Yes, through **three or more** methods.
2 = The program promotes participation in a variety of community physical activity options, but through only **one or two** methods.
1 = The program promotes participation in **only one** type of community physical activity option.
0 = The program does not promote participation in community physical activity options, **or** there is no physical education program.

PA.11 Certified or licensed physical education teachers

Are all **physical education** classes taught by teachers who are **certified or licensed** to teach physical education?

3 = Yes, **all** are.
2 = **Most** classes are.
1 = **Some** classes are.
0 = **No** classes are, **or** there are no physical education classes.

PA.12/A.1 Address special health care needs

Does the **physical education** program consistently use all or most of the following practices as appropriate to include students with **special health care needs**?

✓ Encouraging active participation; modifying type, intensity, and length of activity if indicated in Individualized Education Plans, asthma action plans, or **504 plans**

✓ Offering adapted physical education classes

✓ Using modified equipment and facilities

✓ Ensuring that students with **chronic health conditions** are fully participating in physical activity as appropriate and when able

✓ Monitoring signs and symptoms of chronic health conditions

✓ Encouraging students to carry and self-administer their medications (including pre-medicating and/or responding to asthma symptoms) in the gym and on playing fields; assisting students who do not self-carry

✓ Encouraging students to actively engage in self-monitoring (i.e., using a peak flow meter, recognizing triggers) in the gym and on playing fields (if the parent/guardian, health care provider, and school nurse so advise)

✓ Using a second teacher, aide, physical therapist, or occupational therapist to assist students, as needed

✓ Using peer teaching (e.g., teaming students without special health care needs with students who have such needs)

3 = Yes, the physical education program uses **all or most** of these instructional practices consistently.

2 = The physical education program uses **some** of these instructional practices consistently.

1 = The physical education program uses **some** of these instructional practices, **but** not consistently (that is, not by all teachers or not in all classes that include students with special health care needs).

0 = The program uses **none** of these practices, **or** there is no physical education program.

PA. 13/S.1/A.2 Physical education safety practices

Does the **physical education** program implement and enforce all of the following safety practices?
- ✓ Practice **active supervision**
- ✓ Encourage **pro-social behaviors**
- ✓ Use protective clothing and safety gear that is appropriate to child's size and in good shape
- ✓ Use safe, age-appropriate equipment
- ✓ Minimize exposure to sun (including through use of sunscreen), smog, and extreme temperatures
- ✓ Use infection control practices for handling blood and other body fluids
- ✓ Monitor the environment to reduce exposure to potential allergens or irritants (e.g., pollen, bees, strong odors)

3 = Yes, **all** these safety practices are followed.

2 = All these safety practices are followed, **but** at times our school has temporary lapses in implementing or enforcing one of them.

1 = One of these safety practices is not followed, **or** at times our school has temporary lapses in implementing or enforcing more than one of them.

0 = More than one of these safety practices is not followed, **or** there is no physical education program.

PA.14/S.2 Playgrounds meet safety standards

Does your school or district ensure that playgrounds meet or exceed recommended safety standards for design, installation, and maintenance, in all of the following ways?

✓ Using recommended safety surfaces under playground equipment
✓ Using developmentally-appropriate equipment designed with spaces and angles that preclude entrapment
✓ Designating boundaries around equipment (e.g., swings) so that students on foot are unlikely to be struck
✓ Separating playgrounds from motor vehicle and bicycle traffic
✓ Maintaining equipment for safe use and removing unsafe equipment
✓ Ensuring that **staff members** are trained in developmental appropriateness of different types of playground equipment
✓ Developing, implementing, and enforcing rules for safe use of the playground (e.g., no running or pushing, no use of age-inappropriate equipment)

NOTE: Please disregard any standard that is not relevant for your campus.

3 = Yes, **all** these safety standards are met.
2 = **All** these safety standards are met, **but** at times our school has temporary lapses in implementing or enforcing one of them.
1 = One of these safety standards is not met, **or** at times our school has temporary lapses in implementing or enforcing more than one of them.
0 = More than one of these safety standards is not met, **or** there are no playgrounds.

PA.15   Professional development for teachers

Are teachers of **physical education** required to participate at least once a year in **professional development** in physical education?

3 = Yes, **all** do.
2 = **Most** do.
1 = **Some** do.
0 = **None** do, **or** no one teaches physical education.

PA.16   Participation in intramural programs or physical activity clubs

Do both boys and girls participate in school-sponsored **intramural programs or physical activity clubs**?

3 = Yes, **many** boys and girls participate in school-sponsored intramural programs or physical activity clubs.
2 = For the most part, many students of **only one sex** participates in school-sponsored intramural programs or physical activity clubs.
1 = **Very few** students of either sex participate in school-sponsored intramural programs or physical activity clubs.
0 = There are **no** school-sponsored intramural programs or physical activity clubs.

PA.17 Promotion or support of walking and bicycling to school

Does your school promote or support walking and bicycling to school in the following ways?
✓ Designation safe or preferred routes to school
✓ Promotional activities such as participation in International Walk to School Week
✓ Storage facilities for bicycles and helmets

3 = Yes, our school promotes or supports walking and bicycling to school in all **three** of these ways.
2 = Our school promotes or supports walking and bicycling to school in **two** of these ways.
1 = Our school promotes or supports walking and bicycling to school in **one** of these ways.
0 = Our school does **not** promote or support walking and bicycling to school.

PA. 18/S.3 Physical activity facilities meet safety standards

Does the school ensure that spaces and facilities for physical activity meet or exceed recommended safety standards for design, installation, and maintenance, in the following ways?

✓ Regular inspection and repair of indoor and outdoor playing surfaces, including those on playgrounds and sports fields
✓ Regular inspection and repair of physical activity equipment such as balls, jump ropes, nets, cardiovascular machines, weights, and weight lifting machines
✓ Padded goal posts and gym walls
✓ Breakaway bases for baseball and softball
✓ Securely anchored portable soccer goals that are stored in a locked facility when not in use
✓ Bleachers that minimize the risk for falls
✓ Slip-resistant surfaces near swimming pool use
✓ Pools designed, constructed, and retrofitted to eliminate entrapment use

NOTE: Please disregard any standard that is not relevant for your campus.

3 = Yes, all these safety standards are met.
2 = All these safety standards are met, **but** at times the school has temporary lapses in one of them.
1 = One of these safety standards is not met, **or** at times the school has temporary lapses in more than one of them.
0 = More than one of these safety standards is not met, **or** there are no spaces or facilities for physical activity.

Module 3: Physical Education and Other Physical Activity Programs

Planning Questions
(photocopy before using)

The Module 3 Planning Questions will help your school use its School Health Index results to identify and prioritize changes that will improve policies and programs to improve students' health and safety.

Planning Question 1
Look back at the scores you assigned to each question. According to these scores, what are the **strengths** and the **weaknesses** of your school's physical education and other physical activity policies and programs?

Planning Question 2
For each of the weaknesses identified above, list several recommended actions to improve the school's scores (e.g., provide 150 minutes of physical education per week).

Continued on next page

SCHOOL HEALTH INDEX – ELEMENTARY SCHOOL

Planning Question 3. List each of the actions identified in Planning Question 2 on the table below. Use the five-point scales defined below to rank each action on five dimensions (importance, cost, time, commitment, feasibility). Add the points for each action to get the total points. Use the total points to help you choose one, two, or three top priority actions that you will recommend to the School Health Index team for implementation this year.

Importance	How important is the action to my school?		
	5 = Very important	3 = Moderately important	1 = Not important
Cost	How expensive would it be to plan and implement the action?		
	5 = Not expensive	3 = Moderately expensive	1 = Very expensive
Time	How much time and effort would it take to implement the action?		
	5 = Little or no time and effort	3 = Moderate time and effort	1 = Very great time and effort
Commitment	How enthusiastic would the school community be about implementing the action?		
	5 = Very enthusiastic	3 = Moderately enthusiastic	1 = Not enthusiastic
Feasibility	How difficult would it be to complete the action?		
	5 = Not difficult	3 = Moderately difficult	1 = Very difficult

Module 3 Actions	Importance	Cost	Time	Commitment	Feasibility	Total Points	Top Priority Action?

Module 4: Nutrition Services

Instructions for Module Coordinator

Habits and practices related to health and safety are influenced by the entire school environment. That's why the School Health Index has eight different modules, which correspond to the eight components of coordinated school health in the figure below.

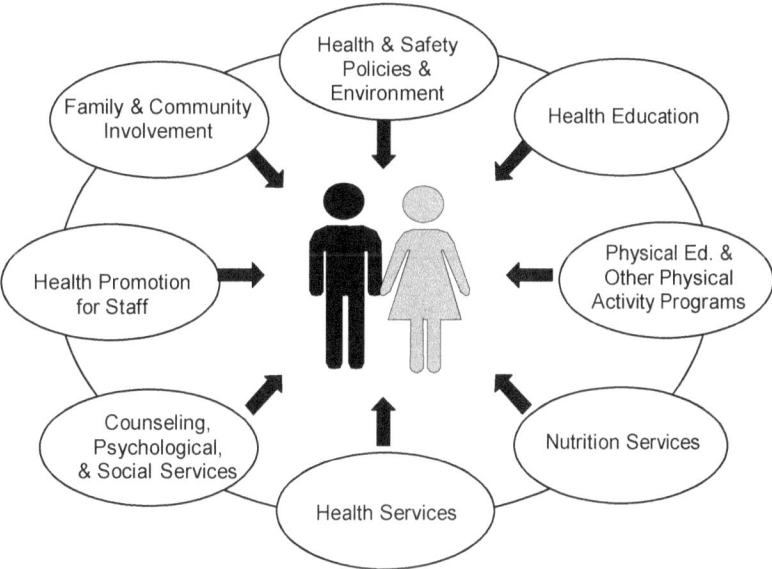

Instructions for completing the module

1. Work with the site coordinator to organize a team to complete the module's documents. Below are some suggested members of the Module 4 team.

School nutrition services manager	Teacher(s)
School nutrition services staff member(s)	Parent(s)
School nurse	Student(s)
Health educator(s)	Assistant principal

2. Make a photocopy of the module Discussion Questions (pages 5-9) for each Module 4 team member. Make at least one photocopy of the module Score Card (page 3) and the module Planning Questions (pages 11-12).

3. Give each Module 4 team member a copy of the Module 4 Discussion Questions. Use the copies of the module Score Card and the Planning Questions to record the team's work. Put the originals of these documents away in case you need to make more photocopies.

4. At a Module 4 team meeting:
   - Discuss each of the Module 4 Discussion Questions and its scoring choices.
   - Decide how to collect any information you need to answer each question accurately.
   - After you have all the information you need, arrive at a consensus score for each question. Answer each question as accurately as possible. The School Health Index is **your** self-assessment tool for identifying strengths and weaknesses and for planning improvements; it should not be used for evaluating staff.
   - Record the scores (0-3) for each question on the module Score Card and calculate the overall Module Score.
   - Use the scores written on the module Score Card to complete the Planning Questions at the end of the module.
   - Use the results from the third Planning Question to identify the one, two, or three highest priority actions that you will recommend to the School Health Index team for implementation this year.
   - Use the answers to the Planning Questions to decide how you will present your results and recommendations at the follow-up School Health Index team meeting.

We wish you success in your efforts to improve the health and safety of young people!

Module 4: Nutrition Services

Score Card
(photocopy before using)

Instructions

1. Carefully read and discuss the Module 4 Discussion Questions (pages 5-9), which contains questions and scoring descriptions for each item listed on this Score Card.
2. Circle the most appropriate score for each item.
3. After all questions have been scored, calculate the overall Module Score and complete the Module 4 Planning Questions located at the end of this module (pages 11-12).

		Fully in Place	Partially in Place	Under Develop-ment	Not in Place
N.1	Breakfast and lunch programs	3	2	1	0
N.2	Variety of foods in school meals	3	2	1	0
N.3	Healthy food purchasing and preparation practices				
N.4	A la carte offerings include healthy food and beverage items	3	2	1	0
N.5	Sites outside cafeteria offer healthy food and beverage items	3	2	1	0
N.6	Promote healthy food and beverage choices	3	2	1	0
N.7	Adequate time to eat school meals	3	2	1	0
N.8	Collaboration between nutrition services staff members and teachers	3	2	1	0
N.9	Degree and certification of nutrition services manager	3	2	1	0
N.10	Professional development for nutrition services manager	3	2	1	0
N.11/ S.1	Clean, safe, pleasant cafeteria	3	2	1	0
N.12/ S.2	Preparedness for food emergencies	3	2	1	0

COLUMN TOTALS: For each column, add up the numbers that are circled and enter the sum in this row.

(If you decide to skip any of the topic areas, make sure you adjust the denominator for the Module Score (36) by subtracting 3 for each question eliminated).

TOTAL POINTS: Add the four sums above and enter the total to the right.

MODULE SCORE = (Total Points / 36) X 100   %

This page intentionally left blank.

Module 4: Nutrition Services

Discussion Questions

N.1 Breakfast and lunch programs

Does your school offer **school meals** (breakfast and lunch) programs that are **fully accessible** to all students?

3 = Yes.
2 = Our school offers breakfast and lunch programs, **but** they are not fully accessible to all students.
1 = Our school offers only a lunch program, **but** there are plans to add a breakfast program.
0 = Our school offers only a lunch program and there are no plans to add a breakfast program, **or** the school does not offer a breakfast or a lunch program.

N.2 Variety of foods in school meals

Do **school meals** include a variety of foods that meet the following criteria?
✓ Go beyond the National School Lunch Program requirements to offer one additional serving per week from any of the 3 vegetable subgroups (dark green, red and orange, dry beans and peas)
✓ Offer a different fruit every day of the week during lunch (100% fruit juice can be counted as a fruit only once per week)
✓ Serve fresh fruit at least 1 day/week
✓ Ensure that at least two-thirds of grains offered each week are **whole grain rich**
✓ Offer at least 3 different types of whole grain-rich foods each week
✓ Offer only nonfat (flavored or unflavored) and **low-fat** (unflavored) fluid milk each day (This is a new requirement of the National School Lunch Program)

Breakfast
✓ Offer at least 3 different fruits and vegetables each week
✓ Serve fresh at least 1 fruit per week
✓ Ensure that at least 50% of grains offered per week are whole grain rich
✓ Offer only nonfat (flavored or unflavored) and **low-fat** (unflavored) fluid milk each day

NOTE: A school meal is a set of foods that meets school meal program regulations. This does not include **à la carte offerings**.

3 = Yes, meets **7-10** of these criteria for variety.
2 = Meets **4-6** of these criteria.
1 = Meets **1-3** of these criteria.
0 = Meets **none** of these criteria.

N.3 Healthy food purchasing and preparation practices

Does the school food service consistently follow all of these food purchasing and preparation practices to reduce the fat and sodium content of foods served?
- ✓ Spoon solid fat from chilled meat and poultry broth before use
- ✓ Use specifications requiring lower fat content in ordering prepared foods such as hamburgers, pizza, chicken nuggets, etc.
- ✓ Rinse browned meat with hot water to remove grease before adding to other ingredients
- ✓ Remove skin from poultry before or after cooking
- ✓ Roast, bake, or broil meat rather than fry it
- ✓ Roast meat and poultry on rack so fat will drain
- ✓ Use low-fat or reduced-fat cheese on pizza
- ✓ Prepare vegetables using little or no fat
- ✓ Cook with nonstick spray or pan liners rather than with grease or oil
- ✓ Offer low-fat salad dressings
- ✓ Use frozen vegetables or low-sodium canned vegetables, instead of regular canned vegetables
- ✓ Use standardized recipes that are low in fats, oils, salt and sugars
- ✓ Use other seasonings in place of salt

3 = Yes, follows all **thirteen** of these practices.
2 = Follows **nine to twelve** of these practices.
1 = Follows **six to eight** of these practices.
0 = Follows **five or fewer** of these practices.

N.4 A la carte offerings include healthy food and beverage items

Do **à la carte offerings** include at least one of each of the following types of food items every day?
- ✓ Fruits or non-fried vegetables
- ✓ Whole grain products (such as whole wheat breads, rolls or bagels; whole wheat pasta; brown rice; whole grain cereals; or rolled oats)
- ✓ Nonfat or **low-fat** dairy products

3 = Yes, à la carte offerings include at least one item from each of these **three** food groups every day **or** no à la carte is offered.
2 = Include at least one item from **two** of these food groups every day.
1 = Include at least one item from **one** of these food groups every day.
0 = Daily à la carte offerings do **not** include items from any of these three food groups.

N.5   Sites outside cafeteria offer healthy food and beverage items

Do most or all <u>**sites outside the cafeteria**</u> where food is available offer fruits, non-fried vegetables, whole grains or nonfat or <u>**low-fat**</u> dairy products?

3 = Yes, **most or all** sites outside the cafeteria do.
2 = **About half** the sites do.
1 = **Fewer than half** the sites do.
0 = **None** of the sites do.

N.6   Promote healthy food and beverage choices

Are food and beverage choices that are low in fat, sodium, and added sugars promoted through the following methods?
✓ Place in more prominent positions than <u>**less nutritious**</u> choices
✓ Offer at competitive prices compared with less nutritious choices
✓ Display nutritional information about available foods
✓ Display promotional materials such as posters
✓ Highlight healthy cafeteria selections in menus that are distributed or posted
✓ Offer taste-testing opportunities
✓ Make school-wide audio or video announcements
✓ Have contests (e.g., recipe competitions)
✓ Engaging students in deciding what foods and beverages are offered

3 = Yes, promoted through **five or more** of these methods.
2 = Promoted through **three or four** of these methods.
1 = Promoted through **one or two** of these methods.
0 = Promoted through **none** of these methods.

N.7   Adequate time to eat school meals

Do students have at least 10 minutes to eat breakfast and at least 20 minutes to eat lunch, counting from the time they are seated?

3 = Yes. (NOTE: If the school does not have a breakfast program, but does provide at least 20 minutes for lunch, you can select 3.)
2 = Have adequate time for breakfast or lunch, but not for both.
1 = No, but there are plans to increase the time.
0 = No.

N.8   Collaboration between nutrition services staff members and teachers

Do nutrition services staff members use three or more of the following methods to collaborate with teachers to reinforce nutrition education lessons taught in the classroom?
- ✓ Participate in design and implementation of nutrition education programs
- ✓ Display educational and informational materials that reinforce classroom lessons
- ✓ Provide food for use in classroom nutrition education lessons
- ✓ Provide ideas for classroom nutrition education lessons
- ✓ Teach lessons or give presentations to students
- ✓ Provide cafeteria tours for classes

3 = Yes, use **three or more** methods.
2 = Use **two** of these methods.
1 = Use **one** of these methods.
0 = Use **none** of these methods.

N.9   Degree and certification of nutrition services manager

Does the school's nutrition services manager have a nutrition-related baccalaureate or graduate degree and certification/credentialing in nutrition services from either the state or the School Nutrition Association?

3 = Yes, has a degree and certification/credentialing.
2 = Has a degree or certification/credentialing, **but** not both.
1 = Has neither a degree nor certification/credentialing, **but** she/he is working on one or both.
0 = Has neither a degree nor certification, **and** she/he is not working on either.

N.10   Professional development for nutrition services manager

Does the nutrition services manager participate at least once a year in **professional development** on both of the following topics?
- ✓ Meeting the Dietary Guidelines for Americans (e.g., meal planning, recipe modification and substitutions, food purchasing and preparation practices)
- ✓ Nutrition education to promote healthy eating choices

3 = Yes.
2 = Participates for one topic, **but** not for the other.
1 = No, **but** there are plans to participate in the near future.
0 = No, **and** there are no plans to participate in the near future.

N.11/S.1 Clean, safe, pleasant cafeteria

Does the school provide students with a clean, safe, and pleasant cafeteria, according to the following criteria?
- ✓ Physical structure (e.g., walls, floor covering) does not need repairs
- ✓ Tables and chairs are not damaged and are of appropriate size for all students
- ✓ Seating is not overcrowded (i.e., never more than 100% of capacity)
- ✓ Rules for safe behavior (e.g., no running, no throwing food or utensils) are enforced
- ✓ Tables and floors are cleaned between lunch periods or shifts
- ✓ Age-appropriate decorations are used
- ✓ Appropriate practices are used to prevent excessive noise levels (e.g., no whistles)
- ✓ Smells are pleasant and not offensive
- ✓ Appropriate eating devices are available when needed for students with **special health care needs**

3 = Yes, cafeteria meets all **nine** of these criteria.
2 = Meets **five to eight** of these criteria.
1 = Meets **three or four** of these criteria.
0 = Meets **two or fewer** of these criteria.

N.12/S.2 Preparedness for food emergencies

Are school nutrition service staff members and cafeteria monitors (e.g., teachers, aides) trained to respond quickly and effectively to the following types of food emergencies?
- ✓ Choking
- ✓ Natural disasters (e.g., electrical outages affecting refrigeration)
- ✓ Medical emergencies (e.g., severe food allergy reactions, diabetic reactions)
- ✓ Attempts to introduce biological or other hazards into the food supply
- ✓ Situations that require students or others to shelter in the school

3 = Yes, trained for all **five** types of emergencies.
2 = Trained for **three or four** types of emergencies.
1 = Trained for **one or two** types of emergencies.
0 = Trained for **none** of these types of emergencies.

This page intentionally left blank.

Module 4: Nutrition Services

Planning Questions
(photocopy before using)

The Module 4 Planning Questions will help your school use its School Health Index results to identify and prioritize changes that will improve policies and programs to improve students' health and safety.

Planning Question 1
Look back at the scores you assigned to each question. According to these scores, what are the **strengths** and the **weaknesses** of your school's food service policies and programs?

Planning Question 2
For each of the weaknesses identified above, list several recommended actions to improve the school's scores (e.g., offer an accessible school breakfast program).

Continued on next page

SCHOOL HEALTH INDEX – ELEMENTARY SCHOOL

Planning Question 3. List each of the actions identified in Planning Question 2 on the table below. Use the five-point scales defined below to rank each action on five dimensions (importance, cost, time, commitment, feasibility). Add the points for each action to get the total points. Use the total points to help you choose one, two, or three top priority actions that you will recommend to the School Health Index team for implementation this year.

Importance	How important is the action to my school?
	5 = Very important 3 = Moderately important 1 = Not important
Cost	How expensive would it be to plan and implement the action?
	5 = Not expensive 3 = Moderately expensive 1 = Very expensive
Time	How much time and effort would it take to implement the action?
	5 = Little or no time and effort 3 = Moderate time and effort 1 = Very great time and effort
Commitment	How enthusiastic would the school community be about implementing the action?
	5 = Very enthusiastic 3 = Moderately enthusiastic 1 = Not enthusiastic
Feasibility	How difficult would it be to complete the action?
	5 = Not difficult 3 = Moderately difficult 1 = Very difficult

Module 4 Actions	Importance	Cost	Time	Commitment	Feasibility	Total Points	Top Priority Action?

Module 5: School Health Services

Instructions for Module Coordinator

Habits and practices related to health and safety are influenced by the entire school environment. That's why the School Health Index has eight different modules, which correspond to the eight components of coordinated school health in the figure below.

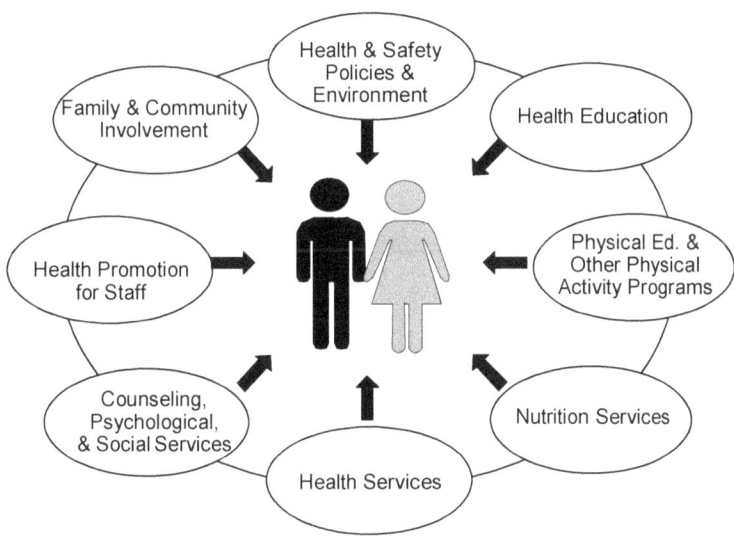

Instructions for completing the module

1. Work with the site coordinator to organize a team to complete the module's documents. Below are some suggested members of the Module 5 team.

School nurse	Assistant principal
Parent(s)	Community-based health care provider
Student(s)	Health department representative(s)
	Counselor(s)

2. Make a photocopy of the module Discussion Questions (pages 5-10) for each Module 5 team member. Make at least one photocopy of the module Score Card (page 3) and the module Planning Questions (pages 11-12).

3. Give each Module 5 team member a copy of the Module 5 Discussion Questions. Use the copies of the module Score Card and the Planning Questions to record the team's work. Put the originals of these documents away in case you need to make more photocopies.

4. At a Module 5 team meeting:
   - Discuss each of the Module 5 Discussion Questions and its scoring choices.
   - Decide how to collect any information you need to answer each question accurately.
   - After you have all the information you need, arrive at a consensus score for each question. Answer each question as accurately as possible. The School Health Index is **your** self-assessment tool for identifying strengths and weaknesses and for planning improvements; it should not be used for evaluating staff.
   - Record the scores (0-3) for each question on the module Score Card and calculate the overall Module Score.
   - Use the scores written on the module Score Card to complete the Planning Questions at the end of the module.
   - Use the results from the third Planning Question to identify the one, two, or three highest priority actions that you will recommend to the School Health Index team for implementation this year.
   - Use the answers to the Planning Questions to decide how you will present your results and recommendations at the follow-up School Health Index team meeting.

We wish you success in your efforts to improve the health and safety of young people!

Module 5: School Health Services

Score Card

Instructions

1. Carefully read and discuss the Module 5 Discussion Questions (pages 5-10), which contains questions and scoring descriptions for each item listed on this Score Card.
2. Circle the most appropriate score for each item.
3. After all questions have been scored, calculate the overall Module Score and complete the Module 5 Planning Questions located at the end of this module (pages 11-12).

		Fully in Place	Partially in Place	Under Develop-ment	Not in Place
CC.1	Health services provided by a full-time school nurse	3	2	1	0
CC.2	Health and safety promotion for students and families	3	2	1	0
CC.3	Collaborate with other school staff members	3	2	1	0
CC.4	Identify and track students with chronic health conditions	3	2	1	0
CC.5	Implement a referral system	3	2	1	0
CC.6	Student health information	3	2	1	0
CC.7	Consulting school health physician	3	2	1	0
S.1	Assess extent of injuries on school property	3	2	1	0
S.2/ A.1	Emergency response plans	3	2	1	0
A.2	Case management for students with poorly controlled asthma	3	2	1	0
A.3	Ensure immediate and reliable access to quick-relief medications for students with asthma	3	2	1	0
A.4	Offer asthma management education to all students with asthma	3	2	1	0

COLUMN TOTALS: For each column, add up the numbers that are circled and enter the sum in this row.

(If you decide to skip any of the topic areas, make sure you adjust the denominator for the Module Score (36) by subtracting 3 for each question eliminated).

TOTAL POINTS: Add the four sums above and enter the total to the right.

MODULE SCORE =
(Total Points / 36) X 100   %

This page intentionally left blank.

Module 5: School Health Services

Discussion Questions

CC.1   Health services provided by a full-time school nurse

Does your school have a **full-time**, registered school nurse **responsible** for **health services** all day, every day? Are an adequate number of full-time school nurses provided, based on the recommended ratio of at least one nurse for every 750 students?

NOTE: More nurses are recommended if students have extensive nursing needs.

3 = Yes, we have a school nurse present all day every day, **and** the recommended ratio is present.
2 = We have a school nurse present all day every day, but **fewer** than one for every 750 students.
1 = We have a school nurse present **some** of the time each week, **or** we have an LPN or UAP (supervised by a school nurse) who is present at least **some** of the time each week.
0 = No, we do **not** have a school nurse, LPN, or UAP present in our school, **or** we have an **unsupervised** LPN or UAP in our school.

CC.2   Health and safety promotion for students and families

Does the school nurse or other **health services provider** promote the health and safety of students and their families, through classroom activities and otherwise, on each of these topics?
✓ Promoting physical activity
✓ Promoting healthy eating
✓ Preventing tobacco use
✓ Quitting tobacco use
✓ Preventing unintentional injuries
✓ Preventing violence and suicide
✓ Managing asthma
✓ Preventing HIV, other STD, and unintended pregnancy

3 = Yes, addresses all **eight** of these topics.
2 = Addresses **four to seven** of these topics.
1 = Addresses **one to three** of these topics.
0 = Addresses **none** of these topics, or the school does not have a school nurse or other health services provider.

CC.3 Collaborate with other school staff members

Does the school nurse or other **health services provider** collaborate with other school **staff members** to promote student health and safety in at least six of the following ways?
- ✓ Developing plans to address student health problems (e.g., **individual health care plans, individual education plans, 504 plans, school team plans**)
- ✓ Providing **professional development**
- ✓ Developing policy
- ✓ Identifying, revising or developing curricula or units/lessons
- ✓ Developing and implementing school-wide and classroom activities
- ✓ Developing School Improvement Plans
- ✓ Establishing communication systems with other school staff

3 = Yes, there is collaboration in **at least six** of these ways.
2 = There is collaboration in **three to five** of these ways.
1 = There is collaboration in **one or two** of these ways.
0 = No, there is **no** collaboration, **or** the school does not have a school nurse or other health services provider.

CC.4 Identify and track students with chronic health conditions

Does the school nurse or other **health services provider** have a system for **identifying and tracking** students with **chronic health conditions**?

3 = Yes, there is a system to identify and track students with chronic health conditions.
2 = Students are systematically identified, **but** not systematically tracked.
1 = Students are identified **only** when an urgent need related to their condition arises at school.
0 = No, there is no system for identifying or tracking students with chronic health conditions, **or** the school does not have a school nurse or other health services provider.

CC.5 Implement a referral system

Does your school implement a systematic approach (including the following components) for referring students, as needed, to appropriate school- or community-based **health services**?

✓ Contact parents of students identified as potentially needing additional health services and recommend that the students be evaluated by their primary health care provider or specialist.

✓ Contact parents of students without a primary health care provider and give information about child health insurance programs and primary care providers.

✓ Referral information is distributed widely (e.g., through flyers, brochures, website, student handbook, health education class) so that students, staff, and families can learn about school and community services without having to contact school staff.

✓ **Staff members** are given clear guidance on referring students to school **counseling, psychological and social services**.

✓ Referral forms are easy for staff members to access, complete, and submit confidentially.

✓ A designated staff person (e.g., school nurse, counselor) regularly reviews and sorts referral forms and conducts initial screening.

✓ With written parental permission, additional information (e.g., questionnaires, relevant records, brief testing) is gathered as necessary and in compliance with **FERPA**.

✓ Written consent is obtained, in compliance with **HIPAA**, to gather relevant records from other professionals or agencies, if applicable.

✓ A list is kept and regularly updated of youth-friendly referral providers along with basic information about each (e.g., cost, location, language, program features, previous client feedback)

✓ Meetings are held with all relevant parties to discuss referral alternatives.

✓ Potential barriers (e.g., cost, location, transportation, stigma) and how to overcome them are discussed.

✓ Follow-up (e.g., via telephone, text messaging, email, personal contact) is conducted to evaluate the referral and gather feedback about the service.

✓ A status report is provided to the person who identified the problem, if applicable and in compliance with FERPA and/or HIPAA.

✓ **Professional development** is provided to all staff members about the referral process.

3 = Yes, our school has a referral system that includes **all** of these components.
2 = Our school has a referral system that includes **many** of these components.
1 = Our school has a referral system that includes a **few** of these components.
0 = Our school's referral system does **not** include any of these components, **or** our school does not have a referral system.

CC.6 Student health information

Does your school have a system for collecting student health information prior to school entry and every year thereafter? Is **all pertinent information** communicated **in writing** to all **appropriate staff members**?

3 = Yes, all pertinent information is systematically collected and communicated **in writing** to **all** appropriate staff members.
2 = All pertinent information is systematically collected and communicated to **some, but not all** appropriate staff members.
1 = **Some** pertinent information is collected and communicated to **some** staff members.
0 = Pertinent information is **not** collected.

CC.7 Consulting school health physician

Does your school have access to and work with a **consulting school health physician** who assists with your school health programs?

3 = Yes, our school has access to a consulting school health physician **and** has worked with him/her within the past year.
2 = Our school has access to a consulting school health physician through our state or local education or health agency **and** has worked with him/her within the past **two** years.
1 = Our school has access to a consulting school health physician through our state or local education or health agency but has **not** worked with him/her within the past **two** years.
0 = No, our school does **not** have access to a consulting school health physician.

S.1   Assess extent of injuries on school property

Does the school nurse or other **health services provider** systematically collect **information** on unintentional injuries and violence that occur on school property (including school buses) or that are associated with school-sponsored events? Is the information analyzed and consistently reviewed by school policy-makers?

3 = Yes, information is collected, analyzed, and consistently reviewed by school policy-makers.
2 = Information is collected, analyzed, and occasionally reviewed by school policy-makers.
1 = Information is collected and analyzed **but** not reviewed by school policymakers.
0 = Information is collected but not analyzed or reviewed, **or** information is not collected, **or** the school does not have a school nurse or other health services provider.

S.2/A.1   Emergency response plans

Does the school nurse or other **health services provider** have an emergency plan that includes all the components listed below for assessing, managing, and referring students and **staff members** suffering from a medical emergency (e.g., injury, severe asthma episode) to the appropriate level of care?
✓ Written instructions on contacting emergency service providers, with telephone numbers posted in prominent locations
✓ List of health services and other staff members and their assignments, including at least one qualified person who will assess the person(s) suffering from a medical emergency and manage immediate care; one person who will call emergency medical services (EMS); one person who will control students in the area; and one person who will direct EMS to the location of the person(s) suffering from a medical emergency
✓ Multiple methods for accessing EMS
✓ Plan for transporting and referring person(s) suffering from a medical emergency to care, including a protocol for situations in which staff members need to be with a student at a treatment center
✓ System for contacting parents and **appropriate staff members** (e.g., a central file with daytime contact information for parents and guardians)
✓ Provisions for obtaining parental consent if referral for immediate treatment is required
✓ Copies of treatment and referral protocols available in first aid kits

3 = Yes, **all** of these components are part of the emergency plan.
2 = **All but one** of these components are part of the emergency plan.
1 = There is a plan, **but** it lacks more than one of these components.
0 = No, the school does **not** have a plan.

A.2 Case management for students with poorly controlled asthma

Does your school **facilitate** or provide **case management** for students with **poorly controlled asthma**?

3 = Yes, case management is facilitated or provided to **all** students with poorly controlled asthma.
2 = Case management is facilitated or provided to **most** students with poorly controlled asthma.
1 = Case management is facilitated or provided to **some** students with poorly controlled asthma.
0 = No, case management is **not** facilitated or provided to students with asthma.

A.3 Ensure immediate and reliable access to quick-relief medications for students with asthma

Does your school use all of these methods to ensure all students with asthma have immediate and reliable access to quick-relief medications in school?
✓ Allow students to carry and self-administer quick-relief medications with written permission from physician, parent/guardian, and school nurse.
✓ Ensure quick-relief medication is readily accessible, clearly labeled, and not accessible to other students.
✓ Ensure that someone trained in administering quick-relief asthma medications is always present at the school (e.g., school nurse, health assistant, other school staff).

3 = Yes, students are allowed to carry and self-administer quick-relief medications.
2 = Quick-relief medication is readily accessible, clearly labeled, and not accessible to other students **and** someone trained in administering quick-relief medications is always present at the school.
1 = Quick-relief medication is readily accessible, clearly labeled, and not accessible to other students **or** someone trained in administering quick-relief medications is always present at the school.
0 = No, **none** of these methods are used.

A.4 Offer asthma management education to all students with asthma

Does your school **offer asthma management education** at school for all students with known asthma?

3 = Yes, our school offers asthma management education for **all** students with known asthma
2 = Our school offers asthma management education for **most** students with known asthma.
1 = Our school offers asthma management education for **some** students with known asthma.
0 = No, our school does **not** offer asthma management education for students with known asthma.

Module 5: School Health Services

Planning Questions
(photocopy before using)

The Module 5 Planning Questions will help your school use its School Health Index results to identify and prioritize changes that will improve policies and programs to improve students' health and safety.

Planning Question 1
Look back at the scores you assigned to each question. According to these scores, what are the **strengths** and the **weaknesses** of your school's health services related to students' health and safety?

Planning Question 2
For each of the weaknesses identified above, list several recommended actions to improve the school's scores (e.g., implement a system to refer students to community-based health services).

Continued on next page

Planning Question 3. List each of the actions identified in Planning Question 2 on the table below. Use the five-point scales defined below to rank each action on five dimensions (importance, cost, time, commitment, feasibility). Add the points for each action to get the total points. Use the total points to help you choose one, two, or three top priority actions that you will recommend to the School Health Index team for implementation this year.

Importance	**How important is the action to my school?**		
	5 = Very important	3 = Moderately important	1 = Not important
Cost	**How expensive would it be to plan and implement the action?**		
	5 = Not expensive	3 = Moderately expensive	1 = Very expensive
Time	**How much time and effort would it take to implement the action?**		
	5 = Little or no time and effort	3 = Moderate time and effort	1 = Very great time and effort
Commitment	**How enthusiastic would the school community be about implementing the action?**		
	5 = Very enthusiastic	3 = Moderately enthusiastic	1 = Not enthusiastic
Feasibility	**How difficult would it be to complete the action?**		
	5 = Not difficult	3 = Moderately difficult	1 = Very difficult

Module 5 Actions	Importance	Cost	Time	Commitment	Feasibility	Total Points	Top Priority Action?

Module 6: School Counseling, Psychological, and Social Services

Instructions for Module Coordinator

Habits and practices related to health and safety are influenced by the entire school environment. That's why the School Health Index has eight different modules, which correspond to the eight components of coordinated school health in the figure below.

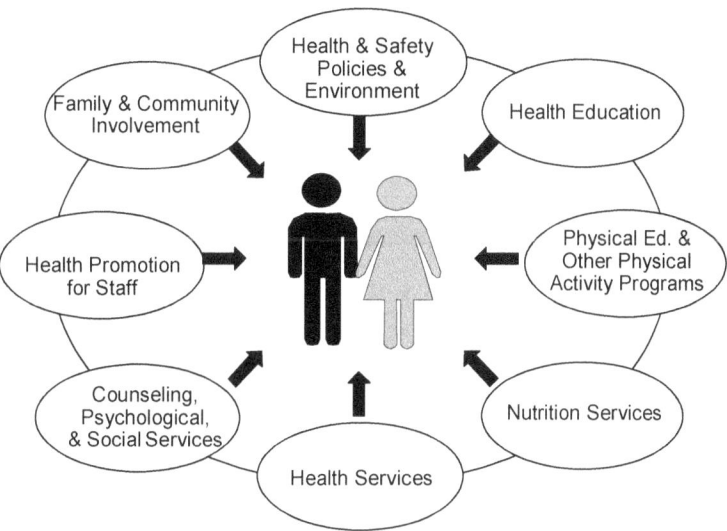

Instructions for completing the module

1. Work with the site coordinator to organize a team to complete the module's documents. Below are some suggested members of the Module 6 team.

School counselor	Parent(s)
School psychologist	Student(s)
School social worker	Community-based social services provider
School nurse	Health care provider
Assistant principal	Special education team leader

2. Make a photocopy of the module Discussion Questions (pages 5-9) for each Module 6 team member. Make at least one photocopy of the module Score Card (page 3) and the module Planning Questions (pages 11-12).

3. Give each Module 6 team member a copy of the Module 6 Discussion Questions. Use the copies of the module Score Card and the Planning Questions to record the team's work. Put the originals of these documents away in case you need to make more photocopies.

4. At a Module 6 team meeting:
    - Discuss each of the Module 6 Discussion Questions and its scoring choices.
    - Decide how to collect any information you need to answer each question accurately.
    - After you have all the information you need, arrive at a consensus score for each question. Answer each question as accurately as possible. The School Health Index is **your** self-assessment tool for identifying strengths and weaknesses and for planning improvements; it should not be used for evaluating staff.
    - Record the scores (0-3) for each question on the module Score Card and calculate the overall Module Score.
    - Use the scores written on the module Score Card to complete the Planning Questions at the end of the module.
    - Use the results from the third Planning Question to identify the one, two, or three highest priority actions that you will recommend to the School Health Index team for implementation this year.
    - Use the answers to the Planning Questions to decide how you will present your results and recommendations at the follow-up School Health Index team meeting.

We wish you success in your efforts to improve the health and safety of young people!

Module 6: School Counseling, Psychological, and Social Services

Score Card
(photocopy before using)

Instructions

1. Carefully read and discuss the Module 6 Discussion Questions (pages 5-9), which contains questions and scoring descriptions for each item listed on this Score Card.
2. Circle the most appropriate score for each item.
3. After all questions have been scored, calculate the overall Module Score and complete the Module 6 Planning Questions located at the end of this module (pages 11-12).

		Fully in Place	Partially in Place	Under Develop-ment	Not in Place
CC.1	Counseling, psychological, and social services provided by a full-time counselor, social worker, and psychologist	3	2	1	0
CC.2	Health and safety promotion and treatment	3	2	1	0
CC.3	Collaborate with other school staff members	3	2	1	0
CC.4	Identify and track students with emotional, behavioral and mental health needs	3	2	1	0
CC.5	Establish referral system	3	2	1	0
CC.6	Aid students during transitions	3	2	1	0
S.1	Identify and refer students involved in violence	3	2	1	0

COLUMN TOTALS: For each column, add up the numbers that are circled and enter the sum in this row.

(If you decide to skip any of the topic areas, make sure you adjust the denominator for the Module Score (21) by subtracting 3 for each question eliminated).

TOTAL POINTS: Add the four sums above and enter the total to the right.

MODULE SCORE =
(Total Points / 21) X 100

%

This page intentionally left blank.

Module 6: School Counseling, Psychological, and Social Services

Discussion Questions

CC.1   Counseling, psychological, and social services provided by a full-time counselor, social worker, and psychologist

Does your school have access to a **full-time** counselor, social worker, and psychologist for providing **counseling, psychological, and social services**? Is an adequate number of these staff members provided based on the following recommended ratios?
- ✓ One counselor for every 250 students
- ✓ One social worker for every 400 students
- ✓ One psychologist for every 1,000 students

3 = Yes, we have a full-time counselor, social worker, and psychologist, **and** the recommended ratios are present.

2 = We have a full-time counselor, social worker, and psychologist, but **fewer** than the recommended ratios.

1 = We have a full-time counselor, social worker **or** psychologist, **but** not all three.

0 = No, we do **not** have even one full-time counselor, social work or psychologist.

CC.2   Health and safety promotion and treatment

Does the **counseling, psychological, or social services** provider promote the **emotional, behavioral, and mental health** of and provide treatment to students and families in the following ways?
- ✓ 1-on-1 counseling/sessions
- ✓ Small group counseling/sessions
- ✓ Classroom-based health promotion and prevention
- ✓ School-wide health promotion and prevention

3 = Yes, it is provided in all four ways.

2 = It is provided in 1-on-1 and small group sessions, **and** classroom-based **or** school-wide activities.

1 = It is provided **only** via 1-on-1 and small group sessions.

0 = No, our counseling, psychological, or social services provider does **not** promote emotional, behavioral, and mental health or provide treatment in any of these ways **or** we do not have such a provider.

CC.3 Collaborate with other school staff members

Does the **counseling, psychological, or social services** provider collaborate with other school **staff members** to promote student health and safety in at least six of the following ways?
- ✓ Developing plans to address student health problems (e.g., **individual health care plans, individual education plans, 504 plans, school team plans**)
- ✓ Providing **professional development**
- ✓ Developing policy
- ✓ Identifying, revising or developing curricula or units/lessons
- ✓ Developing and implementing school-wide and classroom activities
- ✓ Developing School Improvement Plans
- ✓ Establishing communication systems with other school staff

3 = Yes, there is collaboration in **at least six** of these ways.
2 = There is collaboration in **three to five** of these ways.
1 = There is collaboration in **one or two** of these ways.
0 = No, there is **no** collaboration, or the school does **not** have a counseling, psychological, or social services provider.

CC.4 Identify and track students with emotional, behavioral, and mental health needs

Does the **counseling, psychological, or social services** provider have a system for **identifying and tracking** students with **emotional, behavioral, and mental health needs**?

3 = Yes, there is a system to identify and track students with emotional, behavioral, and mental health needs.
2 = Students are systematically identified, **but** not systematically tracked.
1 = Students are identified **only** when an urgent need arises at school.
0 = No, there is **no** system for identifying or tracking students with emotional, behavioral, and mental health needs, **or** the school does not have a counseling, psychological, or social services provider.

CC.5 Establish referral system

Does your school implement a systematic approach (including the following components) for referring students, as needed, to appropriate school- or community-based **counseling, psychological, and social services**?

✓ Case management, including assessment, referral, education, support, and monitoring, is offered.

✓ Referral information is distributed widely (e.g., through flyers, brochures, website, student handbook, health education class) so that students, staff, and families can learn about school and community services without having to contact school staff.

✓ **Staff members** are given clear guidance on referring students to school counseling, psychological, and social services.

✓ Referral forms are easy for staff members to access, complete, and submit confidentially.

✓ A designated staff person (e.g., school counselor, social worker, or psychologist) regularly reviews and sorts referral forms and conducts initial screening.

✓ With written parental permission, additional information (e.g., questionnaires, relevant records, brief testing) is gathered as necessary and in compliance with **FERPA**.

✓ Written consent is obtained, in compliance with **HIPAA**, to gather relevant records from other professionals or agencies, if applicable.

✓ A list is kept and regularly updated of youth-friendly referral providers along with basic information about each (e.g., cost, location, language, program features, previous client feedback, types of insurance accepted)

✓ Meetings are held with all relevant parties to discuss referral alternatives.

✓ Potential barriers (e.g., cost, location, transportation, stigma), and how to overcome them, are discussed.

✓ Follow-up (e.g., via telephone, text messaging, email, personal contact) is conducted to evaluate the referral and gather feedback about the service.

✓ A status report is provided to the person who identified the problem, if applicable and in compliance with FERPA and/or HIPAA.

✓ Professional development is provided to all staff members about the referral process.

3 = Yes, our school has a referral system that includes **all** of these components.
2 = Our school has a referral system that includes **some** of these components.
1 = Our school has a referral system that includes a **few** of these components.
0 = Our school's referral system does **not** include any of these components, **or** our school does not have a referral system.

CC.6 Aid students during transitions

Does your school aid students during school and life transitions (such as changing schools or changes in family structure) in the following ways?
- ✓ Matching new students with another student or buddy
- ✓ Opportunities for students to check-in with a trusted adult
- ✓ Orientation programs that focus on adapting to transitions

3 = Yes, our school aids students during school and life transitions in all **three** of these ways.

2 = Our school aids students during school and life transitions in **two** of these ways.

1 = Our school aids students during school and life transitions in **one** of these ways.

0 = No, our school does **not** aid students during school and life transitions in these ways.

S.1 Identify and refer students involved in violence

Does the **counseling, psychological, or social services** provider have a system for identifying students who have been involved (as a bystander, victim, perpetrator, or some combination of these) in any type of violence (e.g., child abuse, dating violence, sexual assault, **bullying** or **harassment**, fighting, suicide and self-harm behaviors) and, if necessary, refer them to the most appropriate school-based or community-based services?

3 = Yes, identifies and refers students to the most appropriate services.

2 = Identifies and refers students, **but** does not always refer them to the most appropriate services.

1 = Identifies students, **but** sometimes does not refer them to appropriate services.

0 = Does not identify students at risk, **or** the school does not have a counseling, psychological, or social services provider.

This page intentionally left blank.

Module 6: School Counseling, Psychological, and Social Services

Planning Questions
(photocopy before using)

The Module 6 Planning Questions will help your school use its School Health Index results to identify and prioritize changes that will improve policies and programs to improve students' health and safety.

Planning Question 1
Look back at the scores you assigned to each question. According to these scores, what are the strengths and the weaknesses of your school's counseling, psychological, and social services related to students' health and safety?

Planning Question 2
For each of the weaknesses identified above, list several recommended actions to improve the school's scores (e.g., establish a system for referring students to appropriate community-based counseling, psychological, and social services).

Continued on next page

SCHOOL HEALTH INDEX – ELEMENTARY SCHOOL

Planning Question 3. List each of the actions identified in Planning Question 2 on the table below. Use the five-point scales defined below to rank each action on five dimensions (importance, cost, time, commitment, feasibility). Add the points for each action to get the total points. Use the total points to help you choose one, two, or three top priority actions that you will recommend to the School Health Index team for implementation this year.

Importance	**How important is the action to my school?**		
	5 = Very important	3 = Moderately important	1 = Not important
Cost	**How expensive would it be to plan and implement the action?**		
	5 = Not expensive	3 = Moderately expensive	1 = Very expensive
Time	**How much time and effort would it take to implement the action?**		
	5 = Little or no time and effort	3 = Moderate time and effort	1 = Very great time and effort
Commitment	**How enthusiastic would the school community be about implementing the action?**		
	5 = Very enthusiastic	3 = Moderately enthusiastic	1 = Not enthusiastic
Feasibility	**How difficult would it be to complete the action?**		
	5 = Not difficult	3 = Moderately difficult	1 = Very difficult

Module 6 Actions	Importance	Cost	Time	Commitment	Feasibility	Total Points	Top Priority Action?

Module 7: Health Promotion for Staff

Instructions for Module Coordinator

Habits and practices related to health and safety are influenced by the entire school environment. That's why the School Health Index has eight different modules, which correspond to the eight components of coordinated school health in the figure below.

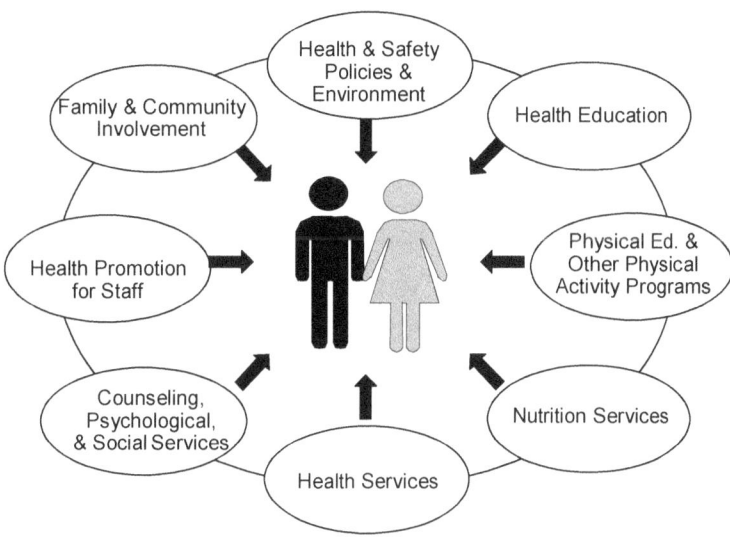

Instructions for completing the module

1. Work with the site coordinator to organize a team to complete the module's documents. Below are some suggested members of the Module 7 team.

Physical education teacher	Community health agency representatives(s)
School nurse	(e.g., American Cancer Society, local health
Teacher(s)	department)
Health educator(s)	Parent(s)
Assistant principal	Community business representative

2. Make a photocopy of the module Discussion Questions (pages 5-11) for each Module 7 team member. Make at least one photocopy of the module Score Card (page 3) and the module Planning Questions (pages 13-14).

3. Give each Module 7 team member a copy of the Module 7 Discussion Questions. Use the copies of the module Score Card and the Planning Questions to record the team's work. Put the originals of these documents away in case you need to make more photocopies.

4. At a Module 7 team meeting:
   - Discuss each of the Module 7 Discussion Questions and its scoring choices.
   - Decide how to collect any information you need to answer each question accurately.
   - After you have all the information you need, arrive at a consensus score for each question. Answer each question as accurately as possible. The School Health Index is **your** self-assessment tool for identifying strengths and weaknesses and for planning improvements; it should not be used for evaluating staff.
   - Record the scores (0-3) for each question on the module Score Card and calculate the overall Module Score.
   - Use the scores written on the module Score Card to complete the Planning Questions at the end of the module.
   - Use the results from the third Planning Question to identify the one, two, or three highest priority actions that you will recommend to the School Health Index team for implementation this year.
   - Use the answers to the Planning Questions to decide how you will present your results and recommendations at the follow-up School Health Index team meeting.

We wish you success in your efforts to improve the health and safety of young people!

Module 7: Health Promotion for Staff

Score Card
(photocopy before using)

Instructions
1. Carefully read and discuss the Module 7 Discussion Questions (pages 5-11), which contains questions and scoring descriptions for each item listed on this Score Card.
2. Circle the most appropriate score for each item.
3. After all questions have been scored, calculate the overall Module Score and complete the Module 7 Planning Questions located at the end of this module (pages 13-14).

		Fully in Place	Partially in Place	Under Develop-ment	Not in Place
CC.1	Health education for staff members	3	2	1	0
CC.2	Health assessments for staff members	3	2	1	0
CC.3	Promote staff member participation	3	2	1	0
CC.4	Stress management programs for staff	3	2	1	0
CC.5	Breastfeeding policy	3	2	1	0
S.1	Training for staff members on conflict resolution	3	2	1	0
S.2	Training for staff members on first aid and CPR	3	2	1	0
PA.1	Programs for staff members on physical activity/fitness	3	2	1	0
N.1	Programs for staff members on healthy eating/weight management	3	2	1	0
T.1	Programs for staff members on tobacco-use cessation	3	2	1	0
A.1	Programs for staff members on asthma management and/or education	3	2	1	0

COLUMN TOTALS: For each column, add up the numbers that are circled and enter the sum in this row.

(If you decide to skip any of the topic areas, make sure you adjust the denominator for the Module Score (33) by subtracting 3 for each question eliminated).

TOTAL POINTS: Add the four sums above and enter the total to the right.

MODULE SCORE =
(Total Points / 33) X 100   %

This page intentionally left blank.

Module 7: Health Promotion for Staff

Discussion Questions

CC. 1 Health education for staff members

Does your school or district **offer staff members** health education and health-promoting activities that focus on skill development and behavior change and that are **tailored** to their needs and interests?

3 = Yes, health education is offered **and** it is tailored to staff members' needs and interests.
2 = Health education is offered and it is tailored to staff members' needs and interests, **but** it does not focus on skill development or behavior change.
1 = Health education is offered, **but** it is not tailored nor does it focus on skill development or behavior change.
0 = No, health education is **not** offered.

CC.2 Health assessments for staff members

Does your school or district **offer staff members** accessible and free or low-cost **health assessments** at least once a year?

3 = Yes, health assessments are offered, and **all** staff members find them accessible and free or low-cost.
2 = Health assessments are offered, but **some** staff members find them inaccessible or high-cost.
1 = Health assessments are offered, but **many** staff members find them inaccessible or high-cost.
0 = Health assessments are **not** offered at least once a year.

CC.3 Promote staff member participation

Does your school or district use three or more **methods to promote and encourage staff member participation** in its health promotion programs?

3 = Yes, uses **three or more** of these methods.
2 = Uses **two** of these methods.
1 = Uses **one** of these methods.
0 = Uses **none** of these methods.

CC.4   Stress management programs for staff

Does your school or district **offer staff members** accessible and free or low-cost stress management programs at least once a year?

3 = Yes, stress management programs are offered, and **all** staff members find them accessible and free or low-cost.

2 = Stress management programs are offered, but **some** staff members find them inaccessible or high-cost.

1 = Stress management programs are offered, but **many** staff members find them inaccessible or high-cost.

0 = Stress management programs are **not** offered at least once a year.

CC.5   Breastfeeding policy

Does your school have a breastfeeding policy that includes the following components?
- ✓ Work schedule flexibility, including breaks and work patterns to provide time for expression of milk
- ✓ Private location to breastfeed or express milk
- ✓ Refrigerator for safe storage of expressed milk
- ✓ Access nearby to a clean, safe water source and a sink for washing hands and rinsing out any breast-pumping equipment

3 = Yes our breastfeeding policy includes all **four** of these components.

2 = Our breastfeeding policy includes **two or three** of these components.

1 = Our breastfeeding policy includes **one** of these components.

0 = Our breastfeeding policy includes **none** of these components, **or** we do **not** have a breastfeeding policy.

S.1   Training for staff members on conflict resolution

Does the school or district **offer staff members** training on conflict resolution that is accessible and free or low-cost?

3 = Yes.
2 = Offers training on conflict resolution, but **some** staff members find it inaccessible or expensive.
1 = Offers training on conflict resolution, but **many** staff members find it inaccessible or expensive.
0 = Does **not** offer training on conflict resolution.

S.2   Training for staff members on first aid and CPR

Does the school or district **offer staff members** training on first aid and cardiopulmonary resuscitation (CPR) that is accessible and free or low-cost?

3 = Yes.
2 = Offers training on first aid and CPR, but **some** staff members find it inaccessible or expensive.
1 = Offers training on first aid and CPR, but **many** staff members find it inaccessible or expensive.
0 = Does **not** offer training on first aid and CPR.

PA.1 Programs for staff members on physical activity/fitness

Does the school or district **offer staff members** accessible and free or low-cost **physical activity/fitness programs**?

3 = Yes.

2 = Offers physical activity/fitness programs, but **some** staff members find them inaccessible or expensive.

1 = Offers physical activity/fitness programs, but **many** staff members find them inaccessible or expensive.

0 = Does **not** offer physical activity/fitness programs.

N.1 Programs for staff members on healthy eating/weight management

Does the school or district **offer staff members** healthy eating/weight management programs that are accessible and free or low-cost?

3 = Yes.
2 = Offers healthy eating/weight management programs, but **some** staff members find them inaccessible or expensive.
1 = Offers healthy eating/weight management programs, but **many** staff members find them inaccessible or expensive.
0 = Does **not** offer healthy eating/weight management programs.

T.1   Programs for staff members on tobacco-use cessation

Does the school or district **offer staff members** tobacco-use **cessation services** that are accessible and free or low-cost?

3 = Yes.
2 = Offers tobacco-use cessation services, but **some** staff members find them inaccessible or expensive.
1 = Offers tobacco-use cessation services, but **many** staff members find them inaccessible or expensive.
0 = Does **not** offer tobacco-use cessation services.

A.1 Programs for staff members on asthma management

Does the school or district **offer staff members** asthma management programs that are accessible and free or low-cost?

3 = Yes.
2 = Offers asthma management programs, but **some** staff members find them inaccessible or expensive.
1 = Offers asthma management programs, but **many** staff members find them inaccessible or expensive.
0 = Does **not** offer asthma management programs.

This page intentionally left blank.

Module 7: Health Promotion for Staff

Planning Questions
(photocopy before using)

The Module 7 Planning Questions will help your school use its School Health Index results to identify and prioritize changes that will improve policies and programs to improve the staff's health and safety.

Planning Question 1
Look back at the scores you assigned to each question. According to these scores, what are the **strengths** and the **weaknesses** of your school's policies and programs related to health promotion for staff?

Planning Question 2
For each of the weaknesses identified above, list several recommended actions to improve the school's scores (e.g., provide easy access to health assessments for staff).

Continued on next page

SCHOOL HEALTH INDEX – ELEMENTARY SCHOOL

Planning Question 3. List each of the actions identified in Planning Question 2 on the table below. Use the five-point scales defined below to rank each action on five dimensions (importance, cost, time, commitment, feasibility). Add the points for each action to get the total points. Use the total points to help you choose one, two, or three top priority actions that you will recommend to the School Health Index team for implementation this year.

Importance	How important is the action to my school?		
	5 = Very important	3 = Moderately important	1 = Not important
Cost	How expensive would it be to plan and implement the action?		
	5 = Not expensive	3 = Moderately expensive	1 = Very expensive
Time	How much time and effort would it take to implement the action?		
	5 = Little or no time and effort	3 = Moderate time and effort	1 = Very great time and effort
Commitment	How enthusiastic would the school community be about implementing the action?		
	5 = Very enthusiastic	3 = Moderately enthusiastic	1 = Not enthusiastic
Feasibility	How difficult would it be to complete the action?		
	5 = Not difficult	3 = Moderately difficult	1 = Very difficult

Module 7 Actions	Importance	Cost	Time	Commitment	Feasibility	Total Points	Top Priority Action?

Module 8: Family and Community Involvement

Instructions for Module Coordinator

Habits and practices related to health and safety are influenced by the entire school environment. That's why the School Health Index has eight different modules, which correspond to the eight components of coordinated school health in the figure below.

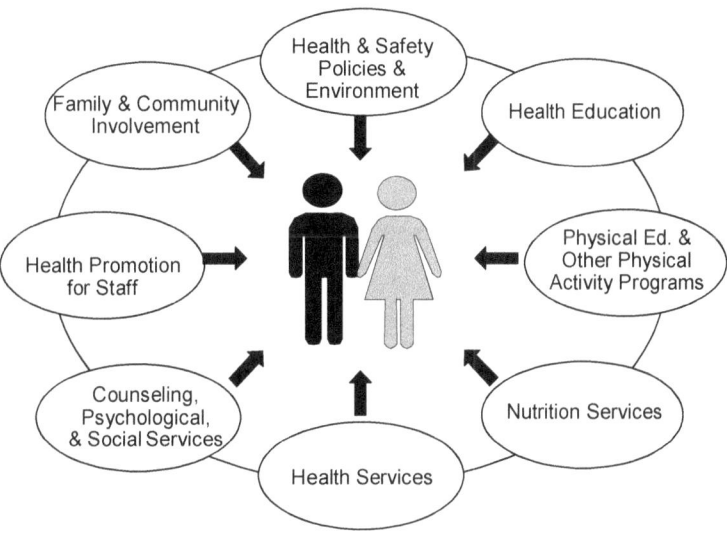

Instructions for completing the module

1. Work with the site coordinator to organize a team to complete the module's documents. Below are some suggested members of the Module 8 team.

Parent(s)	Community health agency representative(s)
Student(s)	(e.g., American Cancer Society, local health
Teacher(s)	department)
School nurse	School counselor
Assistant principal	Local faith-based organization
Community member(s)	representative(s)

2. Make a photocopy of the module Discussion Questions (pages 5-8) for each Module 8 team member. Make at least one photocopy of the module Score Card (page 3) and the module Planning Questions (pages 9-10).

3. Give each Module 8 team member a copy of the Module 8 Discussion Questions. Use the copies of the module Score Card and the Planning Questions to record the team's work. Put the originals of these documents away in case you need to make more photocopies.

4. At a Module 8 team meeting:
    - Discuss each of the Module 8 Discussion Questions and its scoring choices.
    - Decide how to collect any information you need to answer each question accurately.
    - After you have all the information you need, arrive at a consensus score for each question. Answer each question as accurately as possible. The School Health Index is **your** self-assessment tool for identifying strengths and weaknesses and for planning improvements; it should not be used for evaluating staff.
    - Record the scores (0-3) for each question on the module Score Card and calculate the overall Module Score.
    - Use the scores written on the module Score Card to complete the Planning Questions at the end of the module.
    - Use the results from the third Planning Question to identify the one, two, or three highest priority actions that you will recommend to the School Health Index team for implementation this year.
    - Use the answers to the Planning Questions to decide how you will present your results and recommendations at the follow-up School Health Index team meeting.

We wish you success in your efforts to improve the health and safety of young people!

Module 8: Family and Community Involvement

Score Card
(photocopy before using)

Instructions

1. Carefully read and discuss the Module 8 Discussion Questions (pages 5-8), which contains questions and scoring descriptions for each item listed on this Score Card.
2. Circle the most appropriate score for each item.
3. After all questions have been scored, calculate the overall Module Score and complete the Module 8 Planning Questions located at the end of this module (pages 9-10). Be sure to keep your documentation from the small groups to support your recommendations.

		Fully in Place	Partially in Place	Under Develop-ment	Not in Place
CC.1	Communicate with families	3	2	1	0
CC.2	Effective parenting strategies	3	2	1	0
CC.3	Family and community involvement in school decision making	3	2	1	0
CC.4	Family and community volunteers	3	2	1	0
CC.5	Family involvement in learning at home	3	2	1	0
CC.6	Family and community access to school facilities	3	2	1	0
N.1	Student and family involvement in the school meal program	3	2	1	0

COLUMN TOTALS: For each column, add up the numbers that are circled and enter the sum in this row.

(If you decide to skip any of the topic areas, make sure you adjust the denominator for the Module Score (21) by subtracting 3 for each question eliminated).

TOTAL POINTS: Add the four sums above and enter the total to the right.

MODULE SCORE =
(Total Points / 21) X 100

%

This page intentionally left blank.

Module 8: Family and Community Involvement

Discussion Questions

CC.1 Communication with families

Does your school communicate with all families in a **culturally- and linguistically-appropriate** way, using a variety of **communication methods**, about school-sponsored activities and opportunities to participate in school health programs and other **community-based health and safety programs**?

3 = Yes, **all** families are communicated with in a culturally- and linguistically-appropriate way using a variety of communication methods.

2 = **All** families are communicated with using a variety of communication methods, **but** not in a culturally- and linguistically-appropriate way.

1 = Our school only uses very **few** methods to communicate about health-related activities or programs.

0 = Our school does **not** communicate with families in these ways, or families receive communications solely about academic subjects **but** not about health-related activities or programs.

CC.2 Effective parenting strategies

Does your school's family education program address all of the following effective parenting strategies?
✓ Praising and rewarding desirable behavior
✓ Staying actively involved with children in fun activities
✓ Making time to listen and talk with their children
✓ Setting expectations for appropriate behavior and academic performance
✓ Sharing parental values
✓ Communicating with children about health-related risks and behaviors
✓ Making a small number of clear, understandable rules designed to increase level of self-management (e.g., routine household chores, homework, time spent using TV and computer)
✓ Consistently enforcing family rules with consequences (e.g., an additional chore, restricting TV/computer use for the evening)
✓ Monitoring children's daily activities (knowing child's whereabouts and friends)
✓ Modeling nonviolent responses to conflict
✓ Modeling healthy behaviors
✓ Emphasizing the importance of children getting enough sleep
✓ Providing a supportive learning environment in the home

3 = Yes, addresses **all** of these topics.
2 = Addresses **most** of these topics.
1 = Addresses **some** of these topics.
0 = Addresses **none** of these topics, **or** there is no parent education program.

CC.3   Family and community involvement in school decision making

Do families and other community members help with **school decision making**?

3 = Yes, families and community members are actively engaged in **most** school decision-making processes.
2 = Families and community members are actively engaged in **some** school decision-making processes.
1 = Families and community members are offered opportunities to provide input into school decision making **but** are not otherwise engaged.
0 = No, families and community members are **not** engaged in school decision-making processes.

CC.4   Family and community volunteers

Does your school or district have a formal process to recruit, train, and involve family and other community members as **volunteers** to enrich school health and safety programs?

3 = Yes, our school or district has a formal process to recruit, train, and involve parents and other community members.
2 = Our school or district has an informal process to get parents and community members involved.
1 = Our school or district does **not** recruit or train, **but** involves parents and community members when needed.
0 = No, our school or district does **not** recruit, train, or involve parents and community members.

CC.5   Family involvement in learning at home

Does your school provide opportunities for family members to reinforce **learning at home**?

3 = Yes, our school provides family members with opportunities to reinforce learning at home.
2 = Our school provides family members with **limited** opportunities to reinforce learning at home.
1 = Our school provides family members with **very limited** opportunities to reinforce learning at home.
0 = No, our school does **not** provide family members with these opportunities.

CC.6 Family and community access to school facilities

Do family and community members have access to indoor and outdoor school facilities **outside school hours** to participate in or conduct health promotion and education programs?

3 = Yes, community members have access to school facilities.
2 = Community members have **limited** access to school facilities.
1 = Community members have **very limited** access to school facilities, **or** there is access to indoor or outdoor facilities but not to both.
0 = Community members do **not** have access to school facilities.

N.1   Student and family involvement in the school meal program

Do students and family members have opportunities to provide both suggestions for school meals and feedback on the meal program?

3 = Yes, **both** students and family members have opportunities to provide suggestions and feedback.
2 = Yes, **both** students and family members have opportunities to provide **either** suggestions for school meals or feedback on the meal program.
1 = **Either** students or family members have opportunities, **but** not both.
0 = **Neither** students nor family members have these opportunities.

Module 8: Family and Community Involvement

Planning Questions
(photocopy before using)

The Module 8 Planning Questions will help your school use its School Health Index results to identify and prioritize changes that will improve policies and programs to improve students' health and safety.

Planning Question 1
Look back at the scores you assigned to each question. According to these scores, what are the **strengths** and the **weaknesses** of your school's policies and programs related to students' health and safety?

Planning Question 2
For each of the weaknesses identified above, list several recommended actions to improve the school's scores (e.g., increase family education on parenting strategies).

Continued on next page

SCHOOL HEALTH INDEX – ELEMENTARY SCHOOL

Planning Question 3. List each of the actions identified in Planning Question 2 on the table below. Use the five-point scales defined below to rank each action on five dimensions (importance, cost, time, commitment, feasibility). Add the points for each action to get the total points. Use the total points to help you choose one, two, or three top priority actions that you will recommend to the School Health Index team for implementation this year.

Importance	**How important is the action to my school?**		
	5 = Very important	3 = Moderately important	1 = Not important
Cost	**How expensive would it be to plan and implement the action?**		
	5 = Not expensive	3 = Moderately expensive	1 = Very expensive
Time	**How much time and effort would it take to implement the action?**		
	5 = Little or no time and effort	3 = Moderate time and effort	1 = Very great time and effort
Commitment	**How enthusiastic would the school community be about implementing the action?**		
	5 = Very enthusiastic	3 = Moderately enthusiastic	1 = Not enthusiastic
Feasibility	**How difficult would it be to complete the action?**		
	5 = Not difficult	3 = Moderately difficult	1 = Very difficult

Module 8 Actions	Importance	Cost	Time	Commitment	Feasibility	Total Points	Top Priority Action?

Planning for Improvement

Note: Complete this section after all modules have been scored and you are ready to take action.

We all share the same goal: to develop healthy children who come to school ready and able to learn. Among the hundreds of individual actions you can take to meet this goal, you've already begun the most important one – appraising your school's strengths and weaknesses. No matter how your school scores on the SHI, you now have the information you need to start planning for a healthier school.

Taking Action, One Step at a Time

After all eight module teams have completed their sections of the SHI, it is time to summarize the results, reflect on your school's strengths, identify and discuss areas that need improvement, and plan for making improvements.

This section, *Planning for Improvement*, contains two forms, the Overall Score Card and the School Health Improvement Plan, that will help you make the best use of the information collected by each module team.

The four action steps described in this section can help you plan improvements and implement recommended changes.

Step 1:   Complete the Overall Score Card
Step 2:   Complete the School Health Improvement Plan
Step 3:   Implement recommendations
Step 4:   Reassess annually and strive for continuous improvement

Step 1: Complete the Overall Score Card

Use the completed module Score Cards to fill in the Overall Score Card (see page 5 of this section). The completed Overall Score Card will help you determine which of the eight areas covered by the SHI are most in need of improvement. A low score for a module indicates that the school is not performing well in an area, whereas a high score indicates that it is performing well.

Step 2: Complete the School Health Improvement Plan

Bring together the full SHI team for its second meeting. Use the resources, including PowerPoint presentations, provided in the SHI Training Manual to help plan this meeting. (See http://www.cdc.gov/HealthyYouth/SHI/training.) At this meeting:

- Ask each module team to present its self-assessment and the two or three actions they believe should be implemented first.

- Decide on several actions that the school can realistically commit to implementing over the course of the year. Having a relatively small number of recommended actions is important, because pushing for too many changes at once can be overwhelming and reduce your chances of success. Module actions not included in the School Health Improvement Plan can be addressed later.

- The group may consider different criteria in deciding which actions to implement first. Some very important actions may be too expensive, too labor-intensive, or too complex to address in the short term. Others may be less important, but require fewer resources and thus may be easier to implement. It's always a good idea to start with some goals that you are confident can be met in the short term; having some early successes will generate enthusiasm for your efforts. Use the collective judgment and knowledge of your team members. Together, the team knows the school and can arrive at the best mix of important and achievable recommendations.

- Have the team complete the School Health Improvement Plan form (see a sample completed form on page 9) as follows:
  - **Actions column**: Write the agreed-upon actions in order of priority.
  - **Steps column**: Write brief descriptions of all the specific steps that need to be taken to implement an action. Examples of action steps include collecting information on the issue, preparing a slide presentation, making presentations at staff and PTA meetings, scheduling a meeting with the school board, and drafting a new school policy.
  - **By Whom and When column**: Write the name of the person who will be responsible for planning and implementing the action steps and the targeted completion date.

- Decide who will prepare a concise report that summarizes the School Health Improvement Plan, as well as all the recommended actions from all the modules. This report can be presented to the school administrators (or the site decision-making team) for approval and inclusion in the overall School Improvement Plan, and it can guide future school health planning efforts.

- Discuss how the team will monitor implementation of the School Health Improvement Plan and when the team will meet again.

Step 3: Implement Recommendations

When your School Health Improvement Plan has been approved, implement the recommendations and monitor progress. To identify materials and organizations that can help you implement your actions, review the SHI Resources section and the resources available online at www.cdc.gov/HealthyYouth/publications. The online list includes resources for each of the health topics addressed in SHI and for cross-cutting topics such as coordinated school health.

Some actions can be handled quickly and easily by one team member, whereas others may require information gathering, fundraising, or a group effort. A full discussion of project management is beyond the scope of this document, but here are some general principles:

- **Workgroups.** Form implementation workgroups so that no single person is overwhelmed with responsibility.
- **Short-term and long-term goals**. Most positive changes will take some time to put in place, but delayed gratification can be frustrating for many volunteers. Having a mix of short-term and long-term goals creates some early accomplishments that will keep the team motivated while it tackles the longer-term goals.
- **Timeline.** Create a timeline of activities, and set monthly or quarterly implementation milestones.
- **Assistance.** Ask for help when you need it. Look for help from the school district, the state department of education, and local universities.
- **Monitoring progress.** Ongoing monitoring of activities and strategies is essential for smooth and successful implementation. Special achievements and problems should be recognized and discussed.
- **Reporting progress.** Establish a mechanism for reporting progress so that there is some level of accountability.
- **Recognition.** Recognize your volunteers. Write letters of appreciation and publicize their good work so that the entire community will know about their contributions.
- **Money.** If you need money but it is not available at the school, don't be shy about visiting local businesses, especially if you need an amount under $1,000. Write a two-page proposal that uses data, such as the data available for each of the health topics address in the SHI at www.cdc.gov/HealthyYouth/healthtopics.

Step 4: Reassess Annually and Strive for Continuous Improvement

Establish an annual SHI assessment. An annual assessment will ensure that students' health remains high on the school agenda. Take the time to measure and recognize the progress and accomplishments of the previous school year. Report annually to the principal, the superintendent, and the school board on progress made during the past year and plans set for the upcoming year.

This page intentionally left blank.

School Health Index
Overall Score Card

For each module (row), write an X in the one column where the Module Score falls*

	Low 0 – 20%	21% – 40%	Medium 41% – 60%	61% – 80%	High 81% – 100%
School Health Policies and Environment – Module 1					
Health Education – Module 2					
Physical Education and Other Physical Activity Programs – Module 3					
Nutrition Services – Module 4					
School Health Services – Module 5					
School Counseling, Psychological, and Social Services – Module 6					
Health Promotion for Staff – Module 7					
Family and Community Involvement – Module 8					

* Some schools like to write the module scores in each box.

School Health Improvement Plan

Instructions

1. In the first column: list, in priority order, the **actions** that the School Health Index team has agreed to implement.

2. In the second column: list the specific **steps** that need to be taken to implement each action.

3. In the third column: list the people **who** will be responsible for each step and **when** the work will be completed.

Actions	Steps	By Whom and When
1.	a.	
	b.	
	c.	
	d.	
	e.	
	f.	
	g.	

Continued on next page

Actions	Steps	By Whom and When
2.	a. _____ b. _____ c. _____ d. _____ e. _____ f. _____ g. _____	
3.	a. _____ b. _____ c. _____ d. _____ e. _____ f. _____ g. _____	

Actions	Steps	By Whom and When
4.	a.	
	b.	
	c.	
	d.	
	e.	
	f.	
	g.	
5.	a.	
	b.	
	c.	
	d.	
	e.	
	f.	
	g.	

Sample School Health Improvement Plan

Instructions

1. In the first column: list, in priority order, the **actions** that the School Health Index team has agreed to implement.

2. In the second column: list the specific **steps** that need to be taken to implement each action.

3. In the third column: list the people **who** will be responsible for each step and **when** the work will be completed.

Actions	Steps	By Whom and When
1. Establish a set of competitive food offerings that align with strong nutrition standards.	a. Contact other schools and experts to identify different models.	Sally H. 10/2
	b. Conduct taste tests for healthy alternatives that students like.	Mildred P. 10/23
	c. Meet with principal to get support.	Sally H. 10/25
	d. Develop draft competitive food offerings.	Henry T. 11/3
	e. Get feedback from teachers, parents, students, administrators, and community members.	Sally H. 11/15
	f. Develop slide show about new choices to staff, students, parents, and district.	Mildred P. 11/26
	g. Schedule and deliver presentations to staff, students, and parents.	Henry T. 12/2

This page intentionally left blank.

SHI Resources

A comprehensive and up-to-date list of school health and safety resources is available online at www.cdc.gov/HealthyYouth/publications. The online list includes resources for each of the health topics addressed in SHI and for cross-cutting topics such as coordinated school health. Below are some key resources for those modules with cross-cutting questions.

Module 1: School Health and Environment

Improving School Health: A Guide for School Health Councils
http://www.fns.usda.gov/tn/healthy/Ntl_Guide_to_SHAC.pdf
American Cancer Society

Promoting Healthy Youth, Schools, and Communities: A Guide to Community-School Health Advisory Councils
http://www.idph.state.ia.us/hpcdp/common/pdf/family_health/Covers.pdf
Iowa Department of Public Health

School Connectedness: Strategies for Increasing Protective Factors among Youth
http://www.cdc.gov/HealthyYouth/AdolescentHealth/connectedness.htm
Centers for Disease Control and Prevention

Wellness Policy Tool
http://www.actionforhealthykids.org/for-schools/wellness-policy-tool
Action for Healthy Kids

Healthy School Environments Assessment Tool
http://www.epa.gov/schools/healthyseat/index.html
Environmental Protection Agency

National Clearinghouse for Educational Facilities
http://www.ncef.org/
National Institute of Building Sciences

Readiness and Emergency Management for Schools Technical Assistance Center
http://rems.ed.gov/
U.S. Department of Education

Module 2: Health Education

Health Education Curriculum Analysis Tool (HECAT)
http://www.cdc.gov/healthyyouth/hecat/
Centers for Disease Control and Prevention

Health, Mental Health, and Safety Guidelines for Schools: Health and Safety Education
http://www.nationalguidelines.org/chapter_full.cfm?chap=2
Maternal and Child Health Bureau, American Academy of Pediatrics, National Association of School Nurses, American School Health Association, and Centers for Disease Control and Prevention

National Health Education Standards: Achieving Health Literacy
http://www.cdc.gov/healthyyouth/sher/standards/index.htm
Joint Committee on National Health Education Standards

A Competency-based Framework for Health Educators
http://www.ncate.org/LinkClick.aspx?fileticket=J37euHlcN3E%3d&tabid=676
National Council for Accreditation of Teacher Education (NCATE)

Module 5: Health Services

Family Educational Rights and Privacy Act (FERPA)
http://www2.ed.gov/policy/gen/guid/fpco/ferpa/index.html
U.S. Department of Education

Guidelines for Adolescent Preventive Services (GAPS)
http://www.ama-assn.org/ama/pub/physician-resources/public-health/promoting-healthy-lifestyles/adolescent-health/guidelines-adolescent-preventive-services.page
American Medical Association

Module 6: Counseling, Psychological, and Social Services
Family Educational Rights and Privacy Act (FERPA)
http://www2.ed.gov/policy/gen/guid/fpco/ferpa/index.html
U.S. Department of Education

Mental Health in Schools: An Overview
http://smhp.psych.ucla.edu/aboutmh/mhinschools.html
Center for Mental Health in Schools

Module 7: Health Promotion for Staff
School Employee Wellness: A Guide for Protecting the Assets of Our Nation's Schools
http://www.schoolempwell.org
Directors of Health Promotion and Education

Module 8: Family and Community Involvement
Parent Engagement: Strategies for Involving Parents in School Health
http://www.cdc.gov/healthyyouth/adolescenthealth/pdf/parent_engagement_factsheet.pdf
Centers for Disease Control and Prevention

Parent Involvement: Getting Involved
http://www.pta.org/topic_getting_involved.asp
National Parent Teacher Association (PTA)

Positive Parenting Tips
http://www.cdc.gov/ncbddd/childdevelopment/positiveparenting/index.html
Centers for Disease Control and Prevention

Helping Your Child Series
http://www2.ed.gov/parents/academic/help/hyc.html
U.S. Department of Education

This page intentionally left blank.

Glossary

504 plans are written descriptions of educational, health, and other related services or modifications needed to assist students with special needs who are in a regular educational setting.

A la carte offerings means a set of foods from which students can choose individual items that are not usually counted as part of a reimbursable meal.

Actions are steps to take to improve areas you have identified as weaknesses. After analyzing the module scores and using them to identify your school's strengths and weaknesses, you can use the information to brainstorm possible actions for improving the weak areas.

Active learning strategies include interactive teaching methods to encourage student involvement rather than relying solely on a lecture format. Active learning strategies include:
- supervised practice
- discussion
- cooperative learning
- simulations and learning games
- teacher and peer modeling
- role playing
- goal-setting
- rehearsal
- visualization

Actively supervise means using practices such as observing, listening to students, anticipating and effectively responding to unsafe situations, discouraging pushing and bullying, and promoting pro-social behaviors.

All pertinent information is determined in partnership with parents or legal guardians, if possible. All communication should be in compliance with the Family Educational Rights and Privacy Act (FERPA). Communication may be in the form of written mechanisms, such as asthma action plans, allergy alerts, individual health care plans, or injury reports. Regardless of the communication mechanism, pertinent information includes:
- signs or symptoms to watch for in the student
- specific action to take if student exhibits signs or symptoms
- special precautions, if needed
- a reminder about the confidentiality of this information

Appropriate staff members are those who "need to know" and could include: classroom teachers, instructional assistants, physical education teachers, health education teachers, nutrition services staff, school nurses, health assistants, counseling/psychological/social services providers, recess supervisors, coaches, administrators, secretaries, bus drivers, school resource officers, and before- and after-school staff.

Asthma basics and emergency response might include the following topics:
- basic information about asthma, including common asthma triggers, signs and symptoms of asthma
- recognizing and responding to severe asthma symptoms that require immediate action
- the policy permitting students to carry and self-administer prescribed quick relief medications for asthma
- asthma action plans
- eliminating or reducing exposure to asthma triggers
- student health confidentiality
- recognizing and referring signs of poorly controlled asthma

At least 50% of the time means at least half of the total time scheduled for a physical education class session.

Barriers to learning include deficiencies in basic living resources and opportunities for development, psychosocial issues, physical health issues, general stressors, crises and emergencies, difficult transitions associated with stages of schooling, becoming a teen parent, moving to a new school, dealing with homelessness, and adapting to a new culture or customs. Services to address barriers to learning include mental health, special education, nursing, psychological, and social services; counseling; mentoring; tutoring; assistance in the classroom; orientation for new students; and English language acquisition.

Bullying is when one or more students tease, threaten, spread rumors about, hit, shove, or hurt another student over and over again. Bullying can occur in person or through technology. It is not bullying when two students of about the same strength or power argue or fight or tease each other in a friendly way. Anyone can be bullied but those who are perceived as different are more frequently bullied. Some ways in which people are diverse or different include sexual orientation, gender identity, race, color, national origin, sex, religion, appearance, or disability.

Case management is a comprehensive set of services provided by either an individual or a team of medical professionals, school staff, and/or social work staff. These services could include:
- providing referrals to primary healthcare providers
- ensuring an appropriate written asthma action plan is obtained
- ensuring access to and appropriate use of asthma medications, spacers, and peak flow meters at home and at school
- offering asthma education for the student and family
- facilitating environmental modifications at home and at school
- identifying and addressing psychosocial issues related to asthma
- providing additional support services as needed

Certified or licensed means teachers who have been awarded a certificate or license by the state, permitting them to teach physical education.

Cessation services can include any of the following:
- group tobacco-use cessation counseling
- brief clinical counseling
- self-help educational material
- computer-based cessation program
- referral to local physician
- telephone quit line
- pharmacological cessation aid (e.g., nicotine replacement therapy)

Chronic health conditions include asthma, diabetes, overweight/obesity, food allergies, anemia, eating disorders, epilepsy, and oral/dental conditions.

Classroom management techniques might include:
- cooperative learning methods
- social skills training
- promoting interactive learning
- classroom and environmental modification
- conflict resolution and mediation
- behavior management

Commitment is one of the measures used for determining or ranking the priority level of an action. The level of commitment assigned to an action indicates the dedication towards that action by school administration and staff, the community, and you.

Communication methods might include newsletter articles, public access television, website, signs, flyers, phone calls, email, and text messaging.

Community physical activity options might include clubs, teams, recreational classes, special events such as community fun runs, and use of playgrounds, parks, and bike paths.

Community-based health and safety programs might include youth sports and recreation programs; youth development programs; Women, Infants and Children (WIC); food stamps; and activities sponsored by organizations such as YMCA, 4-H programs, Students Against Destructive Decision-Making, Boys and Girls Clubs of America, American Cancer Society, American Heart Association, American Lung Association, and Asthma and Allergy Foundation of America.

Comparable means approximately the same number of students per teacher as in other classes.

Competitive foods and beverages are those outside the federal meal program. They include those offered in vending machines, a la carte, school stores, snack bars, canteens, classroom parties, classroom snacks, school celebrations, fundraisers, or school meetings. These foods are often referred to as competitive foods.

Consistent means that the curriculum addresses the key learning objectives or performance indicators identified by the standards.

Consulting school health physicians support school staff members who are employed to provide physical and mental health services for students and/or staff. He/she has training and/or experience in infant, child, adolescent and/or school health. The physician's function should be specified in a written agreement or contract and may include planning school-based programs, procedures, and protocols; developing health-related school policies; addressing specific health issues of students or staff; or interacting with health professionals in the community on behalf of the school or district.

Coordinator is the facilitator of the SHI process. A coordinator can be someone who is a part of the school or someone external—for example, a retired health educator, community-based dietitian, professor at a local university, graduate student, or a volunteer at a community-based health organization.

Corrective actions are steps that are taken to remove the causes of an existing nonconformity with policy requirements or to make quality improvements. Corrective actions address actual problems. In general, the corrective action process can be thought of as a problem solving process. Examples of a corrective action may include training or professional development.

Cost is one of the measures used for determining or ranking the priority level of an action. The cost indicates the financial resources required to implement an action.

Counseling, Psychological, and Social Services are provided to improve students' mental, emotional, and behavioral health and include individual and group assessments, interventions, and referrals. Organizational assessment and consultation skills of counselors and psychologists contribute not only to the health of students but also to the health of the school environment. Professionals such as certified school counselors, psychologists, and social workers provide these services.

Crisis response plans address environmental disaster (e.g., fire, flood, tornado, blizzard, and earthquake), death or serious injury of a student or staff member, suicide attempt, terrorism, bioterrorism, hazardous chemical spill, explosion, radiation release, mass illness or injury, or any other situation that threatens safety in the school. They include:

- assigned roles and responsibilities for a crisis response team
- procedures for collaborating with local law enforcement and emergency management agencies
- a "go box" containing emergency tools such as: list of students and staff, emergency phone numbers, walkie-talkie system, map and school floor plan, location of power and utility connections
- identification of back-up resources from the district, other schools, and outside groups
- plans for dismissing school early, evacuating students to a safer location, and locking down the building
- designated reunion areas for students and families
- strategy for informing school staff, families, and community about the school's plans
- a media and communications plan
- a plan for screening voluntary offers of assistance
- procedures for handling suspicious packages or envelopes, including actions to minimize exposure to biological and chemical agents
- contact list for grief counselors and other counseling and psychological services
- plans for resuming classes
- evaluating recovery efforts

Cross-cutting questions are questions that apply to all health topic areas and are included in a module regardless of the topics that you select.

Culturally- and linguistically-appropriate means that the materials are appropriate for the intended audience, do not promote biased or stereotypical perceptions of individuals or groups, and are in a language that families can read and understand.

Culturally-appropriate activities and examples include:
- highlighting the contributions and skills of diverse groups of people (e.g., diversity in race, ethnicity, sex, gender identity, sexual orientation, religion, physical or mental ability, appearance, other personal characteristics)
- acknowledging, respecting, and appreciating student diversity
- validating and building students' self-esteem and sense of culture and national background
- strengthening students' skills to engage in intercultural interactions
- not stigmatizing or stereotyping individuals or groups
- building on the cultural resources of families
- featuring diverse groups of people in materials and presentations

Delivery could be addressed through topics such as the following:
- discussion of the curriculum's underlying theory and conceptual framework
- demonstration of program activities by a skilled trainer
- opportunities to practice curricular activities during training
- assessing students' knowledge and skills

Emotional, behavioral, and mental health needs can impact student learning and behavior if not treated or managed. They include diagnosed mental health disorders (for example, Attention Deficit/Hyperactivity Disorder, Anxiety, Bipolar Disorder and Depression) and challenges such as:
- stress, anxiety, and depression
- worries about being bullied
- problems with family or friends
- loneliness or rejection
- disabilities
- thoughts of suicide or hurting others
- concerns about sexuality
- academic difficulties or dropping out
- alcohol, tobacco or other drug use
- inadequate basic life needs (e.g., housing, food, clothing, healthcare)
- pregnancy or parenting
- death of a friend or family member
- addiction
- fear of violence, terrorism or war

Enrichment experiences include athletics, drama, art, music, vocational education, technology training, tutoring services, student clubs, field trips, student advocacy, and community service. These can take place before, during, or after school hours.

Environment is the physical and aesthetic surroundings and the psychosocial climate and culture of the school. Factors that influence the physical environment include the school building and the area surrounding it, any biological or chemical agents that are detrimental to health, and physical conditions such as temperature, noise, and lighting. The psychological environment includes the physical, emotional, and social conditions that affect the well-being of students and staff.

Facilitate means to identify and refer students to case management services.

Family and community involvement is an integrated school, family, and community approach for enhancing the health and well-being of students. School health advisory councils, coalitions, and broadly-based constituencies for school health can build support for school health program efforts. Schools actively solicit family involvement and engage community resources and services to respond more effectively to the health-related needs of students.

Feasibility is one of the measures used for determining or ranking the priority level of an action. The feasibility ranking assigned to an action indicates how likely it is that the school will be able to implement the action.

FERPA, the Family Educational Rights and Privacy Act, is a Federal law that protects the privacy of students' "education records."

Full-time is defined as being present in the school for at least 30 hours per week.

Fully accessible means that the school (1) offers free and reduced-price meals for students who meet income requirement, in a way that ensures these students are not identified by other students as recipients of these programs and (2) coordinates class and bus transportation schedules so that all students can eat breakfast and lunch at school.

Gender expression is how a person publicly expresses their gender to others through appearance and mannerisms (e.g., the way one dresses, talks, acts, moves). A person's gender expression does not necessarily indicate their sexual orientation.

Gender identity is defined as an individual's self-conception as being male or female (or in some cases, both or neither), as distinguished from actual biological sex. For most people, gender identity and biological characteristics are the same. However, some people experience little or no connection between biological sex and gender identity.

Gender roles are the set of activities, expectations and behaviors assigned to females and males based on what a society currently defines as appropriately masculine or feminine.

Harassment is defined under federal civil rights law as conduct based on race, color, national origin, sex, or disability that is so severe, pervasive, or persistent that it creates a hostile environment that interferes or limits a student's ability to participate in or benefit from the services, activities, or opportunities offered by a school. Some state and school district bullying policies go beyond prohibiting bullying on the basis of traits expressly protected by the federal civil rights laws to include sexual orientation, gender identity, and religion. Unlike bullying, harassment does not have to include intent to harm, be directed at a specific person, or involve repeated incidents.

Health assessments might include:
- height and weight
- blood pressure
- cholesterol level
- blood sugar level
- physical activity participation
- dietary habits
- tobacco use
- alcohol and substance use
- safety (e.g., seat belts, helmets, smoke alarms, drinking and driving, coercive or abusive relationships)
- mental health
- confidential HIV counseling, testing, or referral for treatment and care
- sexual health, including testing and treatment for other STD

Health-related fitness means cardiovascular endurance, flexibility, muscular strength, muscular endurance, and body composition.

Health education is a planned, sequential, K-12 curriculum that addresses the physical, mental, emotional, and social dimensions of health. The curriculum is designed to motivate and assist students to maintain and improve their health, prevent disease, and reduce health-related risk behaviors. It allows students to develop and demonstrate increasingly sophisticated health-related knowledge, attitudes, skills, and practices. The comprehensive health education curriculum includes a variety of topics such as personal health, family health, community health, consumer health, environmental health, sexuality education, mental and emotional health, injury prevention and safety, nutrition, prevention and control of disease, and substance use and abuse. Health education is provided by qualified, trained teachers.

Health promotion for staff refers to activities that enable school staff to improve their health status, such as health assessments, health education, and health-related fitness activities. These opportunities encourage school staff to pursue a healthy lifestyle that contributes to their improved health status, improved morale, and a greater personal commitment to the school's overall coordinated health efforts. This personal commitment often transfers into greater commitment to the health of students and creates positive role modeling.

Health services are designed to ensure access or referral to primary health care services or both, foster appropriate use of primary health care services, prevent and control communicable disease and other health problems, provide emergency care for illness or injury, promote and provide optimum sanitary conditions for a safe school facility and school environment, and provide educational and counseling opportunities for promoting and maintaining individual, family, and community health.

Health services providers are qualified professionals such as physicians, nurses, dentists, health educators, and other allied health personnel.

Health topics determine the questions that will be included in your SHI and therefore customize your SHI. The following topics are currently available: safety, physical activity, nutrition, tobacco use, asthma, and sexual health.

HIPAA, the Health Insurance Portability and Accountability Act of 1996 Privacy Rule, requires covered entities to protect individuals' health records and other identifiable health information by requiring appropriate safeguards to protect privacy, and setting limits and conditions on the uses and disclosures that may be made of such information without patient authorization.

HIV, other STD, and pregnancy professional development topics might include:
- describing how widespread teen pregnancy, HIV and other STD infections are and the possible outcomes of these conditions
- understanding the modes of transmission for HIV and other STD and effective prevention strategies for HIV, other STD, and pregnancy
- identifying populations of youth who are disproportionately affected by early pregnancy, HIV, and other STD and the social and behavioral factors that create these disparities
- implementing health education strategies that are likely to be effective in providing youth with the skills to prevent HIV, other STD, and pregnancy
- available evidence-based HIV, other STD, and teen pregnancy prevention programs

Identifying and tracking involves reviewing existing documentation typically collected in schools, such as health history intake forms, emergency contact forms, health room visit logs, incident reports, attendance and early dismissal records, requests for medication administration, calls from school to 911 (or other local emergency numbers), and records of non-participation in physical education and other physical activity. For most chronic health conditions, it does not include screening events or symptom surveys.

Individualized physical activity and fitness plan means a written plan that contains:
- assessment of fitness level (before beginning a new physical activity and fitness plan, individuals should assess their current level of fitness to help avoid injury)
- long-term and short-term personal goals for participating regularly in physical activity and maintaining or improving health-related fitness
- specific actions to achieve those goals
- timeline for taking specific actions, assessing progress, and achieving goals
- methods that will be used to record actions taken and assess progress
- rewards for achieving goals

Information that can be collected on unintentional injuries and violence include:
- date, time, and place of injury
- names of person(s) injured and of any witnesses
- type of injury (e.g., cut, bruise)
- severity of injury (e.g., additional medical care required)
- location of injury (e.g., face, arm)
- activity during which injury occurred (e.g., sporting event, classroom lesson)
- agents of injury (e.g., ball, bat, firearm, knife)
- contributing factors (e.g., alcohol or drug use, lack of supervision, lack of protective gear)
- status of injured person(s) (e.g., student, faculty, staff, visitor)
- relationship of injured party to others (e.g., relative, member of gang)
- intent (e.g., unintentional, assault, self-inflicted)
- description of action taken (e.g., first aid administered, emergency medical services called, parent notified)

Integrate instruction means provide opportunities for students to develop and practice skills in areas such as:
- behavioral skills related to health-related fitness (e.g., self-assessment, goal-setting, decision-making, self-monitoring)
- assessment of health-related fitness (fitness test)
- interpretation and use of fitness test results

Interactions with family members and community organizations include:
- doing homework assignments with parents, guardians, or other family members
- conducting surveys of family members
- sharing information with family members
- exhibiting student projects at school for family viewing
- participating in fun family activities related to safe physical activity and healthy eating
- encouraging family discussion of health topics covered in the classroom
- preparing and practicing safety plans (e.g. home fire escape plan, natural disaster evacuation plan) with the family
- gathering information about existing community-based services
- having students volunteer to help deliver services through community-based organizations, service learning, and community development projects
- participating in community-based special events and attending community-based organizations after school
- participating in community actions such as supporting tobacco-free environments or community gardens
- participating in community advocacy groups (Students Against Destructive Decision-Making, 4-H, and Family, Career, and Community Leaders of America)

Interscholastic sports refer to sports that a school sponsors and are competitive in nature. Examples include:

- baseball
- basketball
- cheerleading or competitive spirits
- cross-country
- fast pitch or slow pitch softball
- field hockey
- football
- golf
- gymnastics
- ice hockey
- lacrosse
- soccer
- swimming or diving
- tennis
- track and field
- volleyball

Intramural programs or physical activity clubs are voluntary in nature (i.e., students have a choice of activities or participation), provide every student an equal opportunity to participate regardless of physical ability, and provide students the opportunity to be involved in planning, organizing, and administering the programs. Examples of intramural activities or physical activity clubs are: open gym days, hiking or walking clubs, dance activities, and tennis clubs.

Learning at home can be encouraged by giving homework assignments that involve family participation; encouraging students to teach their parents about health and safety behaviors; suggesting ways parents can promote healthy behaviors (e.g., picking fruit or hiking); and asking parents to engage their children in health-related learning experiences, such as cooking dinner and packing lunch together, shopping for healthy foods, and reading labels on over-the-counter medicines.

Less nutritious foods and beverages include baked goods and salty snacks that are not low in fat, candy, soda pop, fruit drinks that are not 100% juice, and sports drinks.

Low-fat means either ½% or 1% fat milk.

Meeting the diverse cognitive, emotional, and social needs of children and adolescents might involve:
- organizing and structuring a classroom to promote a positive environment
- using developmentally appropriate discipline strategies that emphasize positive behaviors and values
- effective instruction for diverse learners
- strategies to effectively involve families in children's school life
- strategies to engage students in school and classroom decision making
- strategies to engage English language learners

Methods to promote student participation include:
- class discussions
- bulletin boards
- public address announcements
- guest speakers who promote community programs
- take-home flyers
- homework assignments
- newsletter articles
- academic credit for participating in community physical activities and programs

Methods to promote and encourage staff member participation include:
- information at orientation for new staff members
- information included with paycheck
- flyers posted on school bulletin boards
- letters mailed directly to staff
- announcements at staff meetings
- articles in staff newsletters
- incentive/reward programs
- public recognition
- life/health insurance discounts
- gym or health club discounts, such as YMCA
- posting to a website or listserv
- e-mail messages
- positive role modeling by administrators or other leaders

Moderately to vigorously active means engaging in physical activity that is equal in intensity to or more strenuous than fast walking.

Nutrition services involve access to a variety of nutritious and appealing meals that accommodate the health and nutrition needs of all students. School nutrition programs reflect the U.S. Dietary Guidelines for Americans and other criteria to achieve nutrition integrity. The school nutrition services offer students a learning laboratory for classroom nutrition and health education and serve as a resource for linkages with nutrition-related community services. Qualified child nutrition professionals provide these services.

Offer staff members means that the school or district has arranged for staff members to receive these services either on-site or through a community program off-site. This could be part of the employee benefits package, wellness program, employee assistance program, or through partnership with a community provider.

Offer asthma management education means providing asthma management education, partnering with organizations providing asthma education (e.g., American Lung Association, Asthma and Allergy Foundation of America), providing programming space in school, allowing time for students to participate in school- or community-sponsored programs, or disseminating asthma education materials as a supplement to a formal asthma education program on the following topics:
- basic facts about asthma
- adhering to asthma action plans
- identifying and avoiding triggers
- signs and symptoms of an asthma episode
- medication information
- self-management skills (e.g., monitoring asthma, use of peak flow meter, proper use of inhalers)
- when and how to take emergency actions
- maintaining physical activity

Outside school hours means before and after school and during evenings, weekends, and school vacations.

Pests may include cockroaches, mosquitoes, rats, mice, hornets, ants, spiders, and flies.

Physical activity/fitness programs include classes, workshops, and special events.

Physical education means structured physical education classes or lessons, not physical activity breaks or recess and not substitution of participation in a sport team, ROTC, marching band, etc., for physical education course credit. Physical education is a planned, sequential, K-12 curriculum that provides cognitive content and learning experiences in a variety of activity areas, such as basic movement skills; physical fitness; rhythm and dance; games; team, dual, and individual sports; tumbling and gymnastics; and aquatics. Through a variety of planned physical activities, quality physical education should promote each student's optimum physical, mental, emotional, and social development, including sports that all students enjoy and can pursue throughout their lives. Physical education is provided by qualified trained teachers.

Policies are legal codes, rules, standards, administrative orders, guidelines, mandates, resolutions, or protocols. Policies are usually developed at the school district or state level and implemented at the school level.

Poorly controlled asthma signs include frequent absences from school, frequent visits to the school health office for asthma symptoms, frequent asthma symptoms at school, and/or frequent non-participation in physical education class or physical activity outside of PE class (e.g., recess, after-school physical activity) due to asthma symptoms.

Positive psychosocial school climate is characterized by caring and supportive interpersonal relationships, opportunities to participate in school activities and decision-making, and shared positive norms, goals, and values.

Practices that result in student inactivity include:
- taking attendance while students stand or sit in line
- using games that eliminate students such as dodge ball or elimination tag
- having many students stand in line or on the sidelines watching others and waiting for a turn
- organizing activities in which fewer than half of the students have a piece of equipment and/or a physically active role
- allowing highly skilled students to dominate activities and games

Professional development is the systematic process used to strengthen the professional knowledge, skills, and attitudes of those who serve youth to improve the health, education and well-being of youth. It is consciously designed to actively engage learners and includes the planning, design, marketing, delivery, evaluation, and follow-up of professional development offerings (events, information sessions, and technical assistance).

Prohibit exemptions and waivers means that the school does not allow courses or activities such as interscholastic athletics, ROTC, marching band, cheerleading, or community athletics to be substituted for physical education courses and/or credits.

Punishment should not involve physical activity. Neither punishment nor reward should involve food. For example, schools should prohibit making students run laps or do push-ups as a consequence of inappropriate behavior or not giving one student a snack or meal that is offered to all other students because of inappropriate behavior. Use of food as a reward would include, for example, providing candy or fast-food coupons to students because they have behaved well or met an academic or fundraising goal. Similarly, schools should prohibit withholding of physical education class as a consequence of inappropriate behavior in another class or failure to complete an assignment in another class. (Physical education teachers can discipline students during physical education class by having them sit out for a period of time.)

Recess is an opportunity for unstructured physical activity.

Reference number is a unique number automatically assigned to your team when you register for the online SHI. You will use this number to log in to the system and should save it for future reference.

Representative means that it includes school administrators, health education teachers, physical education teachers, mental health or social services staff members, nutrition services staff members, health services staff members, maintenance and transportation staff members, students, parents, community members, local health departments or organizations, faith-based organizations, businesses, and local government representatives.

Responsible means services are directly provided by the school nurse, or the nurse supervises services provided by licensed practical nurses (LPNs) or unlicensed assistive personnel (UAPs).

School level is the grade level in your school—elementary, middle, or high school. You must choose a school level when creating your SHI.

School meals are school-sponsored or district-sponsored programs that are designed to meet the current U.S. Department of Agriculture (USDA) School Meal Nutrition Standards. As mandated in the Healthy Hunger-Free Kids Act of 2010, the USDA established new meal patterns and nutrition standards for all school meals served in the National School Lunch Program and School Breakfast Program. Key changes include:
- ensuring students are offered both fruits and vegetables every day of the week
- requiring that whole grain-rich foods be offered each week
- offering only fat-free or low-fat milk varieties
- establishing age-appropriate calorie limits for meals
- limiting the amounts of saturated fat, trans fats and sodium

Scorecard is where you mark your scores on the paper version of the SHI. When using the online SHI, your responses to SHI items will be automatically tallied and appear on a scorecard. Module scorecards display your score for the module. The overall scorecard displays your score for all the modules.

Sequential means a curriculum that builds on concepts taught in preceding years and provides opportunities to reinforce skills across topics and grade levels.

SHI name is the name you assigned to your SHI when you created it, for example, LeHigh Health Plan. A SHI name cannot be more than 20 characters long.

Sites outside the cafeteria include:
- vending machines
- school stores and canteens
- concession stands
- parties and special events
- meetings
- extended day programs (i.e., school-sponsored after-school programs)

Skills needed to maintain and improve health include:
- developing critical thinking and problem solving skills
- decision-making and assessing consequences of decisions
- developing communication skills
- developing refusal skills
- expressing feelings in a healthy way
- articulating goals to be healthy
- accessing valid and reliable health information
- identifying and countering health-compromising marketing strategies (e.g., tobacco or alcohol advertising) or media messages (e.g., unprotected sex has no consequences)
- coping with difficult personal situations such as negative peer pressure and family-changes
- managing anger
- building positive relationships
- reading food labels
- planning healthy snacks
- developing a safe, individualized physical activity plan
- wearing and correctly using protective equipment (e.g., bicycle helmet, seat belt, eye protection)

Special health care needs include learning disabilities, developmental disabilities, behavioral disorders, physical disabilities, temporary physical limitations, and chronic medical conditions such as diabetes, asthma, and scoliosis.

Staff members include administrators and clerical workers, classroom teachers, instructional assistants, physical education teachers, health education teachers, aides, nutrition services staff, school nurses, health assistants, counseling/psychological/social services providers, recess supervisors, athletic coaches, facility and maintenance staff, bus drivers, security personnel, volunteers, and before- and after-school staff.

Standard precautions are a set of precautions designed to prevent transmission of human immunodeficiency virus (HIV), hepatitis B virus (HBV), and other bloodborne pathogens when providing first aid or health care, or clean up and disposal of contaminated materials or fluids. Under standard precautions, blood and certain other body fluids of all individuals are considered potentially infectious for HIV, HBV and other bloodborne pathogens.

Strengths are the areas in which you scored high (e.g., 3's and 2's) on your scorecard.

Tailored means that the school or district has conducted a needs assessment to determine which health education topics and health-promoting activities staff members are interested in and what their needs are regarding participation in such activities.

Team is the group of people who will be working on the SHI. The team consists of individuals who are part of the school, such as the principal, students, nurse, parents and teachers; and individuals outside the school, such as local health department staff members.

Team name is the name you assigned to your team, such as LeHigh Tigers. The team name should not exceed 20 characters.

Use of tobacco means all forms both combustible and non-combustible: cigarettes, cigars, cigarillos, chewing tobacco and snuff, bidis, clove cigarettes, etc.

Volunteers might help in the classroom, in the cafeteria, or with special event; lead lunchtime walks, after-school exercise programs, and other health programs; or mentor and tutor students.

Weaknesses are the areas in which you scored low (e.g., 1's and 0's) on your scorecard.

Whole grain rich products are not easily identified because whole grain content is not required on product labels. In practice, the simplest way to determine if a product is whole grain rich is to look at where whole grains appear on the ingredient list. For non-mixed dishes (e.g., breads, cereals), a whole grain must be the primary ingredient by weight (that is, it is the first ingredient in the list.) For mixed dishes (e.g., pizza, corn dogs) a whole grain must be the first grain ingredient in the list.) Detailed instructions for determining if a product is whole grain rich appear in the *HealthierUS School Challenge Whole Grains Resource*, available online.

This page intentionally left blank.